MY COMPLETE PROGRAM NEW COOKBOOK 2024-2025

SAY YES TO QUICK AND FAST 365DAY NUTRITIOUS, FLAVOURFUL RECIPES TO MANAGE, GUIDE, TREAT, TO LOSS YOUR WEIGHT FOR THE FITNESS.

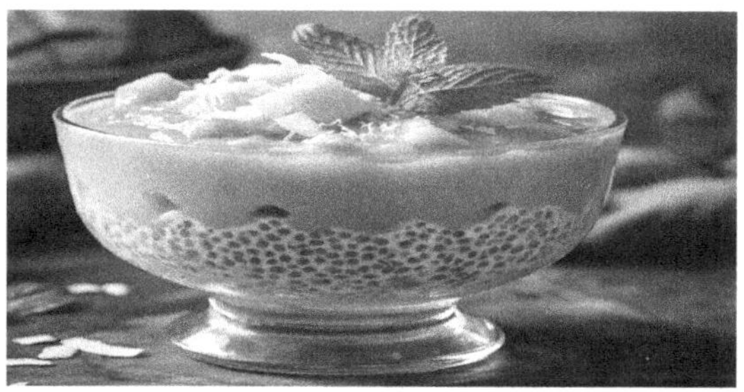

Dr. Godwin James

TABLE OF CONTENT

INTRODUCTION

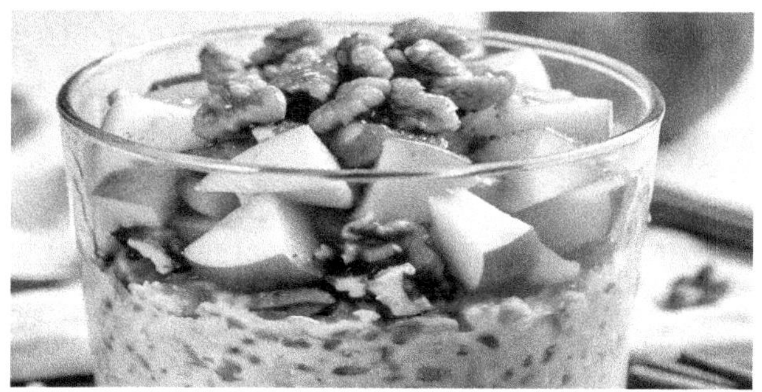

Unlock the Secret to Culinary Bliss - Elevate Every Meal with Nature's Vibrant Treasures!

If you're ready to embark on a journey that will awaken your senses and ignite your passion for cooking, this comprehensive cookbook is your ultimate guide. Prepare to be transported to a world where flavors dance on your tongue, aromas tantalize your soul, and every bite is a celebration of nature's bounty.

Within these pages, you'll discover a treasure trove of recipes that embrace the vibrant hues, rich textures, and intoxicating flavors of the world's most exquisite ingredients. From the verdant greens of sun-kissed fields to the jewel-toned fruits that burst with sweetness, each dish is a masterpiece of color, nutrition, and pure indulgence.

But this cookbook is more than just a collection of recipes – it's a comprehensive program that will empower you to become a true culinary artist. You'll learn time-honored techniques that elevate humble ingredients into extraordinary creations, and gain insights into the art of balancing flavors, textures, and visual appeal.

Imagine starting your day with a vibrant smoothie bowl, a kaleidoscope of nature's finest fruits and superfoods, or savoring a light and refreshing salad bursting with the crisp flavors of the season. As the day unfolds, you'll explore a world of tantalizing main dishes, each one a harmonious fusion of carefully curated ingredients that will leave you feeling nourished and deeply satisfied.

And just when you think the culinary journey has reached its peak, you'll be tempted by a decadent array of desserts that will redefine your understanding of indulgence. From sumptuous cakes and tarts to creamy puddings and velvety mousses, each bite will transport you to a realm of pure bliss.

But this cookbook is more than just a collection of recipes – it's a lifestyle, a celebration of nature's abundance, and a gateway to a world of culinary exploration. With stunning photography and inspiring stories woven throughout, you'll be motivated to embrace a new way of cooking and living, one that honors the earth's gifts and nourishes your body, mind, and spirit.

So, let this cookbook be your guide as you embark on a journey of flavor, wellness, and culinary mastery. Unlock the secrets to creating meals that are not just nourishing but truly soul-stirring, and experience the pure joy of cooking with nature's vibrant treasures.

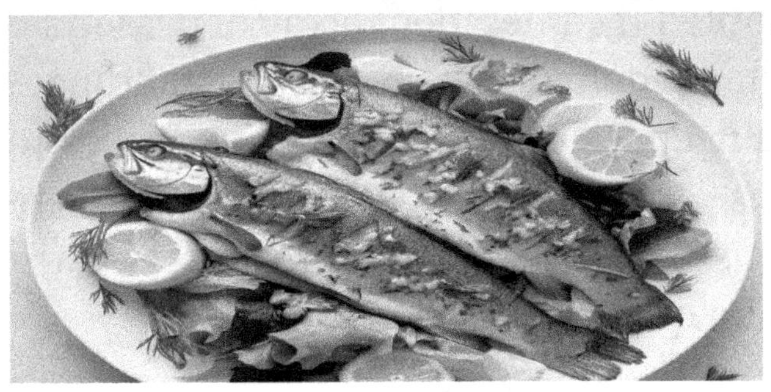

1. Greek Yogurt Parfait

Ingredients:

1 cup non-fat Greek yogurt
1/2 cup fresh berries (strawberries, blueberries, or raspberries)
1 tablespoon honey

2 tablespoons granola (low-sugar)

Instructions:

In a bowl or a glass, layer half of the Greek yogurt.
Add a layer of fresh berries.
Drizzle half the honey over the berries.
Add the remaining Greek yogurt on top.
Sprinkle granola over the top.
Finish with the remaining honey.

(per serving):

Calories: 200
Protein: 15g
Carbohydrates: 35g
Fat: 2g
Fiber: 3g

2. Avocado Toast

Ingredients:

1 slice whole-grain bread

1/2 avocado
1 teaspoon lemon juice
Salt and pepper to taste
Optional: cherry tomatoes, red pepper flakes
Instructions:

Toast the whole-grain bread.
In a small bowl, mash the avocado with lemon juice, salt, and pepper.
Spread the avocado mixture on the toasted bread.
Top with cherry tomatoes and red pepper flakes if desired.

(per serving):

Calories: 200
Protein: 4g
Carbohydrates: 22g
Fat: 12g
Fiber: 7g

3. Veggie Omelet

Ingredients:

2 large eggs
1/4 cup diced bell peppers
1/4 cup diced onions
1/4 cup chopped spinach
Salt and pepper to taste
Cooking spray or 1 teaspoon olive oil
Instructions:

Whisk the eggs in a bowl with salt and pepper.
Heat a non-stick skillet over medium heat and spray with cooking spray or add olive oil.
Sauté the bell peppers and onions until soft, about 3-4 minutes.
Add spinach and cook until wilted, about 1 minute.
Pour the eggs over the vegetables and cook until the edges begin to set, about 2 minutes.
Flip the omelet and cook for another 1-2 minutes until fully cooked.
Serve hot.

(per serving):

Calories: 150
Protein: 12g
Carbohydrates: 5g
Fat: 10g
Fiber: 2g

4. Overnight Chia Pudding

Ingredients:

1/4 cup chia seeds
1 cup unsweetened almond milk
1 teaspoon vanilla extract
1 tablespoon maple syrup
Fresh fruit for topping (optional)
Instructions:

In a mason jar or a bowl, mix chia seeds, almond milk, vanilla extract, and maple syrup.
Stir well to combine.

Cover and refrigerate overnight or for at least 4 hours.
Stir the pudding again before serving.
Top with fresh fruit if desired.

(per serving):

Calories: 200
Protein: 6g
Carbohydrates: 20g
Fat: 11g
Fiber: 10g

5. Banana Oat Pancakes

Ingredients:

1 ripe banana
1/2 cup rolled oats
2 large eggs
1/2 teaspoon baking powder
Cooking spray or 1 teaspoon coconut oil
Optional: a dash of cinnamon, fresh berries for topping
Instructions:

In a blender, combine banana, oats, eggs, and baking powder. Blend until smooth.
Heat a non-stick skillet over medium heat and coat with cooking spray or coconut oil.
Pour small amounts of batter onto the skillet to form pancakes.
Cook until bubbles form on the surface, then flip and cook until golden brown, about 2-3 minutes per side.
Serve with fresh berries if desired.

 (per serving):

Calories: 250
Protein: 12g
Carbohydrates: 35g
Fat: 7g
Fiber: 5g

6. Spinach and Feta Stuffed Breakfast Wrap

Ingredients:

1 whole wheat tortilla (8-inch)
1/2 cup fresh spinach, chopped
1/4 cup crumbled feta cheese
2 large egg whites
Salt and pepper to taste
Cooking spray

Instructions:

Spray a non-stick skillet with cooking spray and heat over medium.
Add spinach and cook until wilted, about 2 minutes.
Add egg whites to the skillet, season with salt and pepper, and scramble until fully cooked.
Remove from heat and stir in feta cheese.
Place the egg mixture in the center of the tortilla, fold in the sides, and roll up to form a wrap.
Serve immediately.

(per serving):

Calories: 220
Protein: 15g
Carbohydrates: 20g
Fat: 10g
Fiber: 3g

7. Berry Smoothie Bowl

Ingredients:

1 cup frozen mixed berries
1/2 banana
1/2 cup unsweetened almond milk
1 tablespoon chia seeds
1 tablespoon almond butter
Toppings: sliced banana, fresh berries, granola (optional)

Instructions:

In a blender, combine frozen berries, banana, almond milk, chia seeds, and almond butter. Blend until smooth.
Pour the smoothie into a bowl.

Top with sliced banana, fresh berries, and a
sprinkle of granola if desired.
Serve immediately.

(per serving):

Calories: 250
Protein: 6g
Carbohydrates: 40g
Fat: 10g
Fiber: 10g

8. Apple Cinnamon Overnight Oats

Ingredients:

1/2 cup rolled oats
1/2 cup unsweetened almond milk
1/4 cup unsweetened applesauce
1/2 teaspoon cinnamon
1 teaspoon maple syrup
Optional: chopped nuts, fresh apple slices
Instructions:

In a mason jar or bowl, mix rolled oats, almond milk, applesauce, cinnamon, and maple syrup.
Stir well to combine.
Cover and refrigerate overnight or for at least 4 hours.
Stir again before serving.
Top with chopped nuts and fresh apple slices if desired.

(per serving):

Calories: 220
Protein: 5g
Carbohydrates: 40g
Fat: 4g
Fiber: 6g

9. Cottage Cheese and Fruit Bowl

Ingredients:

1 cup low-fat cottage cheese
1/2 cup fresh pineapple chunks
1/2 cup fresh strawberries, sliced

1 tablespoon honey
Optional: a sprinkle of cinnamon
Instructions:

In a bowl, combine cottage cheese, pineapple chunks, and sliced strawberries.
Drizzle with honey.
Sprinkle with cinnamon if desired.
Serve immediately.

(per serving):

Calories: 210
Protein: 20g
Carbohydrates: 28g
Fat: 3g
Fiber: 2g

10. Sweet Potato Breakfast Hash

Ingredients:

1 medium sweet potato, peeled and diced
1/2 bell pepper, diced
1/4 red onion, diced

1 large egg
1 teaspoon olive oil
Salt and pepper to taste
Optional: hot sauce

Instructions:

Heat olive oil in a non-stick skillet over medium heat.
Add sweet potato, bell pepper, and red onion. Season with salt and pepper.
Cook, stirring occasionally, until the vegetables are tender and browned, about 10-12 minutes.
Push the vegetables to one side of the skillet and crack the egg into the empty space.
Cook until the egg is done to your liking.
Serve the hash with the egg on top and drizzle with hot sauce if desired.

 (per serving):

Calories: 250
Protein: 8g

Carbohydrates: 35g
Fat: 10g
Fiber: 6g

11. Protein-Packed Smoothie

Ingredients:

1 scoop vanilla protein powder
1 cup unsweetened almond milk
1/2 banana
1 tablespoon peanut butter (natural, no added sugar)
1/2 cup spinach
Ice cubes (optional)

Instructions:

Combine all ingredients in a blender.
Blend until smooth and creamy.
Add ice cubes if desired for a thicker consistency.
Serve immediately.

(per serving):

Calories: 250
Protein: 20g
Carbohydrates: 20g
Fat: 10g
Fiber: 4g

12. Quinoa Breakfast Bowl

Ingredients:

1/2 cup cooked quinoa
1/4 cup low-fat Greek yogurt
1/2 cup mixed berries
1 tablespoon chopped nuts (almonds or walnuts)
1 teaspoon honey
Optional: a sprinkle of cinnamon

Instructions:

Place cooked quinoa in a bowl.
Top with Greek yogurt, mixed berries, and chopped nuts.

Drizzle with honey.
Sprinkle with cinnamon if desired.
Serve immediately.

(per serving):

Calories: 270
Protein: 12g
Carbohydrates: 42g
Fat: 8g
Fiber: 6g

13. Egg Muffins

Ingredients:

4 large eggs
1/2 cup diced bell peppers
1/2 cup diced onions
1/2 cup chopped spinach
Salt and pepper to taste
Cooking spray

Instructions:

Preheat oven to 350°F (175°C).
Spray a muffin tin with cooking spray.
In a large bowl, whisk the eggs with salt and pepper.
Add bell peppers, onions, and spinach to the egg mixture.
Pour the mixture into the muffin tin, filling each cup about 3/4 full.
Bake for 20-25 minutes or until the egg muffins are set and lightly browned.
Allow to cool slightly before removing from the tin.
Serve warm or store in the refrigerator for up to 3 days.

(per serving, 1 muffin):

Calories: 80
Protein: 6g
Carbohydrates: 2g
Fat: 5g
Fiber: 1g

14. Peanut Butter Banana Toast

Ingredients:

1 slice whole-grain bread
1 tablespoon natural peanut butter
1/2 banana, sliced
Optional: a sprinkle of chia seeds or flaxseeds

Instructions:

Toast the whole-grain bread.
Spread peanut butter evenly on the toast.
Top with banana slices.
Sprinkle with chia seeds or flaxseeds if desired.
Serve immediately.

(per serving):

Calories: 210
Protein: 6g
Carbohydrates: 28g
Fat: 9g

Fiber: 5g

15. Cottage Cheese Pancakes

Ingredients:

1/2 cup low-fat cottage cheese
1/4 cup rolled oats
2 large eggs
1/2 teaspoon baking powder
Cooking spray or 1 teaspoon coconut oil
Optional: fresh fruit or a drizzle of honey for topping

Instructions:

In a blender, combine cottage cheese, rolled oats, eggs, and baking powder. Blend until smooth.
Heat a non-stick skillet over medium heat and coat with cooking spray or coconut oil.
Pour small amounts of batter onto the skillet to form pancakes.

Cook until bubbles form on the surface, then flip and cook until golden brown, about 2-3 minutes per side.
Serve with fresh fruit or a drizzle of honey if desired.

(per serving):

Calories: 200
Protein: 16g
Carbohydrates: 18g
Fat: 8g
Fiber: 2g

16. Egg and Avocado Breakfast Sandwich

Ingredients:

1 whole wheat English muffin
1 large egg
1/4 avocado, sliced
1 slice tomato

Salt and pepper to taste
Cooking spray

Instructions:

Split and toast the English muffin.
Spray a non-stick skillet with cooking spray and heat over medium.
Crack the egg into the skillet and cook until the white is set and the yolk is cooked to your liking.
Place the cooked egg on one half of the English muffin.
Top with avocado slices and a slice of tomato.
Season with salt and pepper.
Cover with the other half of the English muffin and serve.

(per serving):

Calories: 250
Protein: 11g
Carbohydrates: 28g

Fat: 12g
Fiber: 6g

17. Blueberry Oatmeal

Ingredients:

1/2 cup rolled oats
1 cup water or unsweetened almond milk
1/2 cup fresh or frozen blueberries
1 teaspoon honey or maple syrup
1/2 teaspoon cinnamon

Instructions:

In a small pot, bring water or almond milk to a boil.
Stir in the oats and reduce heat to a simmer.
Cook for about 5 minutes, stirring occasionally, until the oats are tender.
Stir in the blueberries, honey or maple syrup, and cinnamon.
Serve hot.

(per serving):

Calories: 220
Protein: 6g
Carbohydrates: 40g
Fat: 4g
Fiber: 6g

18. Smoked Salmon and Cucumber Toast

Ingredients:

1 slice whole-grain bread
1 ounce smoked salmon
2 tablespoons light cream cheese
1/4 cucumber, thinly sliced
Fresh dill, for garnish
Lemon juice, to taste
Salt and pepper to taste

Instructions:

Toast the whole-grain bread.
Spread the light cream cheese evenly on the
toast.

Layer the smoked salmon and cucumber slices on top.
Garnish with fresh dill and a squeeze of lemon juice.
Season with salt and pepper.
Serve immediately.

(per serving):

Calories: 200
Protein: 11g
Carbohydrates: 20g
Fat: 9g
Fiber: 3g

19. Mango Chia Pudding

Ingredients:

1/4 cup chia seeds
1 cup unsweetened almond milk
1 teaspoon vanilla extract
1 tablespoon maple syrup
1/2 cup fresh mango, diced
Instructions:

In a mason jar or a bowl, mix chia seeds, almond milk, vanilla extract, and maple syrup.
Stir well to combine.
Cover and refrigerate overnight or for at least 4 hours.
Stir the pudding again before serving.
Top with fresh mango.
Serve immediately.

(per serving):

Calories: 240
Protein: 6g
Carbohydrates: 30g
Fat: 11g
Fiber: 10g

20. Broccoli and Cheese Mini Frittatas

Ingredients:

1 cup broccoli florets, chopped
4 large eggs

1/4 cup shredded cheddar cheese
Salt and pepper to taste
Cooking spray

Instructions:

Preheat oven to 350°F (175°C).
Spray a muffin tin with cooking spray.
Steam or microwave broccoli until tender, then chop finely.
In a large bowl, whisk the eggs with salt and pepper.
Stir in the chopped broccoli and shredded cheddar cheese.
Pour the mixture into the muffin tin, filling each cup about 3/4 full.
Bake for 20-25 minutes or until the frittatas are set and lightly browned.
Allow to cool slightly before removing from the tin.
Serve warm or store in the refrigerator for up to 3 days.
(per serving, 2 mini frittatas):

Calories: 180
Protein: 14g
Carbohydrates: 4g
Fat: 12g
Fiber: 2g

1. Grilled Chicken and Quinoa Salad

Ingredients:

- 1 cup cooked quinoa
- 1 grilled chicken breast, sliced
- 1 cup cherry tomatoes, halved
- 1 cucumber, diced
- 1/4 cup red onion, thinly sliced
- 1/4 cup crumbled feta cheese
- 2 tablespoons chopped fresh parsley
- Juice of 1 lemon
- 1 tablespoon olive oil
- Salt and pepper to taste

Instructions:

1. Prepare Quinoa: Cook quinoa according to package instructions and let it cool.
2. Grill Chicken: Season the chicken breast with salt and pepper. Grill until cooked through and slice into strips.
3. Combine Ingredients: In a large bowl, combine quinoa, chicken, cherry tomatoes, cucumber, red onion, feta cheese, and parsley.
4. Dress Salad: In a small bowl, whisk together lemon juice, olive oil, salt, and pepper. Pour over the salad and toss to combine.
5. Serve: Enjoy this flavorful and filling quinoa salad.

2. Turkey and Avocado Wrap

Ingredients:

- 1 whole wheat tortilla
- 3-4 slices of turkey breast (deli meat)
- 1/2 avocado, sliced
- 1/4 cup shredded lettuce
- 1/4 cup shredded carrots
- 2 tablespoons Greek yogurt
- 1 teaspoon Dijon mustard
- Salt and pepper to taste

Instructions:

1. Prepare Sauce: In a small bowl, mix Greek yogurt and Dijon mustard. Season with salt and pepper.
2. Assemble Wrap: Lay the whole wheat tortilla flat. Spread the yogurt-mustard sauce over the tortilla.
3. Add Fillings: Layer turkey slices, avocado, lettuce, and shredded carrots on top.
4. Wrap: Roll the tortilla tightly, tucking in the sides as you go.

5. Serve: Slice the wrap in half and enjoy.

3. Vegetable Stir-Fry with Tofu

Ingredients:

- 1 block firm tofu, drained and cubed
- 1 tablespoon olive oil
- 2 cups mixed vegetables (bell peppers, broccoli, carrots, snap peas)
- 2 tablespoons low-sodium soy sauce
- 1 tablespoon hoisin sauce
- 1 teaspoon sesame oil
- 1 garlic clove, minced
- 1 teaspoon grated ginger
- 1 cup cooked brown rice

Instructions:

1. Prepare Tofu: Press tofu to remove excess water, then cut into cubes.
2. Cook Tofu: Heat olive oil in a large skillet over medium-high heat. Add tofu cubes and cook until golden brown on all sides. Remove and set aside.
3. Stir-Fry Vegetables: In the same skillet, add garlic and ginger, and sauté for 1 minute. Add mixed vegetables and cook until tender-crisp.
4. Add Sauces: Return tofu to the skillet. Add soy sauce, hoisin sauce, and sesame oil. Stir to combine and cook for another 2-3 minutes.
5. Serve: Serve the stir-fry over cooked brown rice.

4. Spinach and Feta Stuffed Bell Peppers

Ingredients:

- 4 bell peppers, tops cut off and seeds removed
- 1 cup cooked quinoa
- 1 cup fresh spinach, chopped
- 1/2 cup crumbled feta cheese
- 1/4 cup diced red onion
- 1 garlic clove, minced
- 1 tablespoon olive oil
- Salt and pepper to taste

Instructions:

1. Preheat Oven: Preheat your oven to 375°F (190°C).
2. Prepare Filling: In a large bowl, combine cooked quinoa, spinach, feta cheese, red onion, and garlic. Season with salt and pepper.
3. Stuff Peppers: Fill each bell pepper with the quinoa mixture.
4. Bake: Place the stuffed peppers in a baking dish. Drizzle olive oil over the

top. Cover with foil and bake for 30 minutes. Remove foil and bake for an additional 10 minutes until peppers are tender.

5. Serve: Enjoy these nutrient-packed stuffed bell peppers.

5. Tuna and White Bean Salad

Ingredients:

- 1 can (5 oz) tuna in water, drained
- 1 can (15 oz) white beans, drained and rinsed
- 1/2 red onion, finely chopped
- 1/2 cup cherry tomatoes, halved
- 1/4 cup chopped fresh parsley
- Juice of 1 lemon
- 1 tablespoon olive oil
- Salt and pepper to taste

Instructions:

1. Combine Ingredients: In a large bowl, mix together tuna, white beans, red onion, cherry tomatoes, and parsley.
2. Dress Salad: In a small bowl, whisk together lemon juice, olive oil, salt, and pepper. Pour over the salad and toss to combine.
3. Serve: Enjoy this simple, protein-packed salad.

6. Chicken and Veggie Lettuce Wraps

Ingredients:

- 1 lb ground chicken
- 1 tablespoon olive oil
- 1 cup shredded carrots
- 1 cup diced bell peppers
- 1/4 cup diced water chestnuts

- 2 tablespoons low-sodium soy sauce
- 1 tablespoon hoisin sauce
- 1 teaspoon grated ginger
- 1 garlic clove, minced
- Bibb or butter lettuce leaves
- Green onions for garnish

Instructions:

1. Cook Chicken: Heat olive oil in a large skillet over medium-high heat. Add ground chicken and cook until browned, breaking it apart with a spoon.
2. Add Vegetables: Add shredded carrots, bell peppers, water chestnuts, ginger, and garlic. Cook until vegetables are tender.
3. Add Sauce: Stir in soy sauce and hoisin sauce. Cook for an additional 2-3 minutes.

4. Assemble Wraps: Spoon the chicken mixture into lettuce leaves.
5. Serve: Garnish with green onions and serve immediately.

7. Mediterranean Chickpea Salad

Ingredients:

- 1 can (15 oz) chickpeas, drained and rinsed
- 1 cup cherry tomatoes, halved
- 1 cucumber, diced
- 1/4 cup red onion, finely chopped
- 1/4 cup Kalamata olives, pitted and sliced
- 1/4 cup crumbled feta cheese
- 2 tablespoons chopped fresh parsley
- 2 tablespoons olive oil
- Juice of 1 lemon
- Salt and pepper to taste

Instructions:

1. Combine Ingredients: In a large bowl, mix together chickpeas, cherry tomatoes, cucumber, red onion, olives, feta cheese, and parsley.
2. Dress Salad: In a small bowl, whisk together olive oil, lemon juice, salt, and pepper. Pour over the salad and toss to combine.
3. Serve: Enjoy this refreshing and filling salad.

8. Zucchini Noodles with Pesto and Shrimp

Ingredients:

- 2 large zucchinis, spiralized into noodles

- 1 lb shrimp, peeled and deveined
- 1 tablespoon olive oil
- 1/4 cup prepared pesto sauce
- 1/4 cup grated Parmesan cheese
- Salt and pepper to taste

Instructions:

1. Cook Shrimp: Heat olive oil in a large skillet over medium-high heat. Add shrimp and cook until pink and opaque, about 3-4 minutes per side. Remove from skillet and set aside.
2. Cook Zoodles: In the same skillet, add zucchini noodles and cook until tender, about 2-3 minutes.
3. Combine: Return shrimp to the skillet. Add pesto sauce and toss to combine.
4. Serve: Sprinkle with grated Parmesan cheese and serve immediately.

9. **Spinach and Mushroom Quesadilla**

Ingredients:

- 1 whole wheat tortilla
- 1 cup fresh spinach, chopped
- 1/2 cup sliced mushrooms
- 1/4 cup shredded low-fat mozzarella cheese
- 1 tablespoon olive oil
- Salt and pepper to taste

Instructions:

1. Cook Vegetables: Heat olive oil in a skillet over medium heat. Add mushrooms and cook until soft. Add spinach and cook until wilted. Season with salt and pepper.
2. Assemble Quesadilla: Place tortilla in the skillet. Sprinkle half of the cheese

on one half of the tortilla. Add the spinach and mushroom mixture, then top with the remaining cheese. Fold the tortilla over.

3. Cook Quesadilla: Cook until the tortilla is golden brown and the cheese is melted, about 2-3 minutes per side.
4. Serve: Cut into wedges and serve immediately.

10. Tuna and Avocado Salad

Ingredients:

- 1 can (5 oz) tuna in water, drained
- 1 ripe avocado, diced
- 1/2 red bell pepper, diced
- 1/4 cup red onion, finely chopped
- 1 tablespoon fresh lemon juice
- 2 tablespoons chopped fresh cilantro
- Salt and pepper to taste

Instructions:

1. Prepare Ingredients: In a large bowl, combine tuna, avocado, red bell pepper, red onion, lemon juice, and cilantro.
2. Mix Salad: Gently mix until all ingredients are well combined. Season with salt and pepper to taste.
3. Serve: Enjoy as a standalone salad or with whole grain crackers.

DINNER RECIPES

1. Lemon Garlic Baked Salmon

Ingredients:

- 4 salmon fillets (4-6 oz each)
- 2 tablespoons olive oil
- 2 cloves garlic, minced

- Juice of 1 lemon
- Zest of 1 lemon
- 1 teaspoon dried thyme
- Salt and pepper to taste
- Fresh parsley for garnish

Instructions:

1. Preheat Oven: Preheat your oven to 400°F (200°C). Line a baking sheet with parchment paper.
2. Prepare Marinade: In a small bowl, mix together olive oil, minced garlic, lemon juice, lemon zest, dried thyme, salt, and pepper.
3. Marinate Salmon: Place the salmon fillets on the baking sheet. Brush the marinade over the salmon fillets.
4. Bake Salmon: Bake for 12-15 minutes, or until the salmon is cooked through and flakes easily with a fork.

5. Serve: Garnish with fresh parsley and serve with a side of steamed vegetables or a salad.

2. Vegetable Stir-Fry with Brown Rice

Ingredients:

- 1 cup brown rice, cooked
- 2 tablespoons soy sauce (low sodium)
- 1 tablespoon hoisin sauce
- 1 teaspoon sesame oil
- 2 cloves garlic, minced
- 1 teaspoon grated ginger
- 1 cup broccoli florets
- 1 bell pepper, sliced
- 1 cup snap peas
- 1 carrot, sliced
- 1 tablespoon olive oil
- Green onions and sesame seeds for garnish

Instructions:

1. Prepare Rice: Cook brown rice according to package instructions.
2. Make Stir-Fry Sauce: In a small bowl, combine soy sauce, hoisin sauce, and sesame oil.
3. Stir-Fry Vegetables: Heat olive oil in a large skillet over medium-high heat. Add garlic and ginger, and sauté for 1 minute. Add broccoli, bell pepper, snap peas, and carrot. Cook until vegetables are tender-crisp.
4. Add Sauce: Pour the stir-fry sauce over the vegetables and stir to combine. Cook for an additional 2-3 minutes.
5. Serve: Serve the stir-fry over cooked brown rice and garnish with green onions and sesame seeds.

3. Chicken and Vegetable Skewers

Ingredients:

- 2 chicken breasts, cut into 1-inch cubes
- 1 zucchini, sliced
- 1 red bell pepper, cut into squares
- 1 yellow bell pepper, cut into squares
- 1 red onion, cut into squares
- 2 tablespoons olive oil
- 2 tablespoons lemon juice
- 2 cloves garlic, minced
- 1 teaspoon dried oregano
- Salt and pepper to taste
- Wooden skewers (soaked in water for 30 minutes)

Instructions:

1. Preheat Grill: Preheat your grill to medium-high heat.

2. Marinate Chicken: In a bowl, mix together olive oil, lemon juice, garlic, dried oregano, salt, and pepper. Add chicken cubes and vegetables, and toss to coat evenly.
3. Assemble Skewers: Thread the chicken and vegetables onto the skewers, alternating between pieces.
4. Grill Skewers: Grill the skewers for 10-12 minutes, turning occasionally, until the chicken is cooked through and the vegetables are tender.
5. Serve: Serve the skewers with a side salad or whole grain couscous.

4. Spaghetti Squash with Turkey Marinara

Ingredients:

- 1 large spaghetti squash
- 1 lb ground turkey

- 1 tablespoon olive oil
- 1 onion, chopped
- 2 cloves garlic, minced
- 1 can (14.5 oz) diced tomatoes
- 1 can (8 oz) tomato sauce
- 1 teaspoon dried basil
- 1 teaspoon dried oregano
- Salt and pepper to taste
- Fresh basil for garnish

Instructions:

1. Prepare Spaghetti Squash: Preheat your oven to 375°F (190°C). Cut the spaghetti squash in half lengthwise and scoop out the seeds. Place cut-side down on a baking sheet and bake for 35-40 minutes, or until tender. Let cool slightly, then use a fork to scrape out the strands.
2. Cook Turkey: Heat olive oil in a large skillet over medium heat. Add onion

and garlic, and sauté until softened. Add ground turkey and cook until browned.

3. Make Marinara Sauce: Add diced tomatoes, tomato sauce, dried basil, dried oregano, salt, and pepper to the skillet. Simmer for 15-20 minutes.

4. Serve: Serve the turkey marinara sauce over the spaghetti squash strands. Garnish with fresh basil.

5. Stuffed Bell Peppers

Ingredients:

- 4 bell peppers, tops cut off and seeds removed
- 1 lb lean ground beef or turkey
- 1 cup cooked brown rice
- 1 can (14.5 oz) diced tomatoes
- 1/2 onion, chopped
- 2 cloves garlic, minced

- 1 teaspoon dried oregano
- 1 teaspoon dried basil
- Salt and pepper to taste
- 1/2 cup shredded low-fat cheese (optional)

Instructions:

1. Preheat Oven: Preheat your oven to 375°F (190°C).
2. Cook Filling: In a large skillet, cook the ground beef or turkey until browned. Add onion and garlic, and cook until softened. Stir in cooked brown rice, diced tomatoes, oregano, basil, salt, and pepper. Cook for an additional 5 minutes.
3. Stuff Peppers: Fill each bell pepper with the meat and rice mixture. Place them in a baking dish.
4. Bake Peppers: Cover the dish with foil and bake for 30 minutes. If using

cheese, remove foil, sprinkle cheese on top, and bake for an additional 10 minutes until cheese is melted.

5. Serve: Let cool slightly before serving.

6. Cauliflower Fried Rice

Ingredients:

- 1 medium head cauliflower, riced
- 1 tablespoon sesame oil
- 2 cloves garlic, minced
- 1-inch piece ginger, grated
- 1 cup mixed vegetables (carrots, peas, corn)
- 2 eggs, lightly beaten
- 2 green onions, sliced
- 3 tablespoons low-sodium soy sauce
- 1 tablespoon hoisin sauce
- Salt and pepper to taste

Instructions:

1. Prepare Cauliflower: Rice the cauliflower by pulsing florets in a food processor until it resembles rice grains.
2. Cook Vegetables: Heat sesame oil in a large skillet or wok over medium-high heat. Add garlic and ginger, and sauté for 1 minute. Add mixed vegetables and cook until tender.
3. Cook Eggs: Push the vegetables to one side of the skillet. Pour the eggs on the other side and scramble until cooked.
4. Add Cauliflower Rice: Stir in the riced cauliflower and cook for 5-7 minutes until tender.
5. Add Sauce: Stir in soy sauce and hoisin sauce. Mix until well combined and heated through.
6. Serve: Garnish with green onions and serve immediately.

7. **Balsamic Glazed Chicken with Roasted Vegetables**

Ingredients:

- 4 boneless, skinless chicken breasts
- 1/4 cup balsamic vinegar
- 2 tablespoons honey
- 2 cloves garlic, minced
- 1 teaspoon dried thyme
- 1 tablespoon olive oil
- 1 cup cherry tomatoes
- 1 cup baby carrots
- 1 zucchini, sliced
- Salt and pepper to taste

Instructions:

1. Preheat Oven: Preheat your oven to 400°F (200°C).

2. Prepare Marinade: In a small bowl, whisk together balsamic vinegar, honey, garlic, and thyme.

3. Marinate Chicken: Place the chicken breasts in a resealable plastic bag. Pour half of the balsamic mixture over the chicken. Seal the bag and marinate in the refrigerator for at least 30 minutes.

4. Roast Vegetables: On a baking sheet, toss cherry tomatoes, baby carrots, and zucchini with olive oil, salt, and pepper. Roast for 20-25 minutes until tender.

5. Cook Chicken: Heat a large skillet over medium-high heat. Remove chicken from marinade and cook for 6-7 minutes on each side, or until cooked through. Brush with remaining balsamic mixture during the last few minutes of cooking.

6. Serve: Serve the balsamic glazed chicken with the roasted vegetables.

8. **Turkey and Black Bean Enchiladas**

Ingredients:

- 1 lb ground turkey
- 1 can (15 oz) black beans, drained and rinsed
- 1 small onion, chopped
- 1 cup salsa
- 1 tablespoon chili powder
- 1 teaspoon cumin
- 1 cup shredded low-fat cheese
- 8 whole wheat tortillas
- 1 can (10 oz) enchilada sauce
- Fresh cilantro for garnish

Instructions:

1. Preheat Oven: Preheat your oven to 375°F (190°C).

2. Cook Turkey: In a large skillet, cook the ground turkey and onion over medium heat until the turkey is no longer pink. Add black beans, salsa, chili powder, and cumin. Cook for an additional 5 minutes.
3. Assemble Enchiladas: Spoon the turkey mixture down the center of each tortilla. Roll up and place seam-side down in a baking dish. Pour enchilada sauce over the top and sprinkle with cheese.
4. Bake: Cover the dish with foil and bake for 20 minutes. Remove foil and bake for an additional 5-10 minutes until the cheese is melted and bubbly.
5. Serve: Garnish with fresh cilantro and serve.

9. Shrimp and Asparagus Stir-Fry

Ingredients:

- 1 lb shrimp, peeled and deveined
- 1 bunch asparagus, trimmed and cut into 2-inch pieces
- 2 cloves garlic, minced
- 1 tablespoon ginger, minced
- 2 tablespoons soy sauce (low sodium)
- 1 tablespoon oyster sauce
- 1 teaspoon sesame oil
- 1 tablespoon olive oil
- 1 tablespoon cornstarch mixed with 2 tablespoons water (optional for thickening)
- Green onions and sesame seeds for garnish

Instructions:

1. Prepare Shrimp: In a small bowl, combine shrimp with soy sauce, oyster sauce, and sesame oil. Let marinate for 10 minutes.

2. Cook Asparagus: Heat olive oil in a large skillet or wok over medium-high heat. Add asparagus and cook until tender-crisp, about 3-4 minutes. Remove from skillet and set aside.
3. Cook Shrimp: In the same skillet, add garlic and ginger, and sauté for 1 minute. Add shrimp and cook until pink and opaque, about 2-3 minutes per side.
4. Combine: Return asparagus to the skillet. If desired, add cornstarch mixture to thicken the sauce. Cook for an additional 2 minutes until everything is heated through.
5. Serve: Garnish with green onions and sesame seeds. Serve immediately.

10. Zucchini Lasagna

Ingredients:

- 2 large zucchinis, sliced lengthwise into thin strips
- 1 lb lean ground beef or turkey
- 1 cup ricotta cheese (low-fat)
- 1 egg
- 2 cups marinara sauce (low sodium)
- 1 cup shredded mozzarella cheese (low-fat)
- 1/4 cup grated Parmesan cheese
- 1 tablespoon olive oil
- 1 teaspoon dried oregano
- Salt and pepper to taste

Instructions:

1. Preheat Oven: Preheat your oven to 375°F (190°C).
2. Cook Meat: In a large skillet, heat olive oil over medium heat. Add ground beef or turkey, and cook until browned. Add marinara sauce,

oregano, salt, and pepper. Simmer for 10 minutes.

3. Prepare Ricotta Mixture: In a bowl, combine ricotta cheese, egg, salt, and pepper.
4. Assemble Lasagna: In a baking dish, spread a thin layer of meat sauce. Layer zucchini slices over the sauce. Spread a layer of ricotta mixture over the zucchini, then sprinkle with mozzarella cheese. Repeat layers until all ingredients are used, ending with a layer of meat sauce topped with mozzarella and Parmesan cheese.
5. Bake: Cover the dish with foil and bake for 30 minutes. Remove foil and bake for an additional 10-15 minutes until the cheese is melted and bubbly.
6. Serve: Let cool slightly before serving.

FISH AND SEAFOOD RECIPES

1. **Grilled Lemon Herb Salmon**

Ingredients:

- 4 salmon fillets (4 oz each)
- 2 tbsp olive oil
- Juice of 1 lemon
- 2 cloves garlic, minced
- 1 tsp dried oregano
- 1 tsp dried thyme
- Salt and pepper to taste

Instructions:

1. Preheat the grill to medium-high heat.
2. In a small bowl, mix olive oil, lemon juice, garlic, oregano, thyme, salt, and pepper.
3. Brush the salmon fillets with the mixture.
4. Grill the salmon for 5-7 minutes on each side, or until it flakes easily with a fork.
5. Serve immediately with a lemon wedge.

(per serving):

- Calories: 260
- Protein: 23g
- Carbohydrates: 1g
- Fat: 18g
- Fiber: 0g

2. Shrimp and Avocado Salad

Ingredients:

- 1 lb large shrimp, peeled and deveined
- 1 avocado, diced
- 1 cup cherry tomatoes, halved
- 1 cucumber, diced
- 1/4 red onion, thinly sliced
- 2 tbsp fresh lime juice
- 2 tbsp olive oil
- Salt and pepper to taste
- 2 tbsp chopped fresh cilantro

Instructions:

1. Bring a pot of water to a boil. Add shrimp and cook for 2-3 minutes until pink and opaque. Drain and cool.
2. In a large bowl, combine shrimp, avocado, cherry tomatoes, cucumber, and red onion.
3. In a small bowl, whisk together lime juice, olive oil, salt, and pepper.
4. Pour the dressing over the salad and toss gently to combine.
5. Garnish with fresh cilantro before serving.

(per serving):

- Calories: 240
- Protein: 22g
- Carbohydrates: 10g
- Fat: 14g
- Fiber: 5g

3. **Baked Cod with Vegetables**

Ingredients:

- 4 cod fillets (4 oz each)
- 1 zucchini, sliced
- 1 yellow squash, sliced
- 1 red bell pepper, sliced
- 1 tbsp olive oil
- 1 tsp dried basil
- 1 tsp dried oregano
- Salt and pepper to taste
- Juice of 1 lemon

Instructions:

1. Preheat oven to 400°F (200°C).
2. Place cod fillets in a baking dish. Arrange zucchini, yellow squash, and red bell pepper around the fillets.
3. Drizzle olive oil over the fish and vegetables.
4. Sprinkle with basil, oregano, salt, and pepper.

5. Squeeze lemon juice over everything.
6. Bake for 15-20 minutes, or until the fish flakes easily with a fork and vegetables are tender.

(per serving):

- Calories: 180
- Protein: 24g
- Carbohydrates: 6g
- Fat: 6g
- Fiber: 2g

4. Tuna Salad Lettuce Wraps

Ingredients:

- 2 cans (5 oz each) tuna packed in water, drained
- 1/4 cup plain Greek yogurt
- 1 tbsp Dijon mustard
- 1 celery stalk, diced
- 1 small carrot, grated

- 2 green onions, chopped
- Salt and pepper to taste
- 8 large lettuce leaves (e.g., Romaine or butter lettuce)

Instructions:

1. In a medium bowl, mix together tuna, Greek yogurt, Dijon mustard, celery, carrot, green onions, salt, and pepper.
2. Spoon the tuna mixture onto the center of each lettuce leaf.
3. Roll up the lettuce leaves to form wraps.
4. Serve immediately or chill until ready to serve.

(per serving):

- Calories: 110
- Protein: 18g
- Carbohydrates: 3g
- Fat: 3g

- Fiber: 1g

5. Garlic Butter Shrimp Skewers

Ingredients:

- 1 lb large shrimp, peeled and deveined
- 3 tbsp unsalted butter, melted
- 3 cloves garlic, minced
- 1 tbsp fresh parsley, chopped
- 1 tbsp lemon juice
- Salt and pepper to taste
- Skewers (if using wooden skewers, soak them in water for 30 minutes before use)

Instructions:

1. Preheat grill to medium-high heat.
2. In a bowl, combine melted butter, garlic, parsley, lemon juice, salt, and pepper.
3. Thread the shrimp onto the skewers.

4. Brush the shrimp with the garlic butter mixture.
5. Grill the shrimp for 2-3 minutes on each side, or until opaque and cooked through.
6. Serve immediately, garnished with additional parsley if desired.

(per serving):

- Calories: 170
- Protein: 23g
- Carbohydrates: 1g
- Fat: 8g
- Fiber: 0g

6. Blackened Tilapia

Ingredients:

- 4 tilapia fillets (4 oz each)
- 1 tbsp olive oil
- 1 tsp paprika

- 1 tsp garlic powder
- 1 tsp onion powder
- 1/2 tsp cayenne pepper
- 1/2 tsp dried thyme
- 1/2 tsp dried oregano
- Salt and pepper to taste
- Lemon wedges for serving

Instructions:

1. In a small bowl, combine paprika, garlic powder, onion powder, cayenne pepper, thyme, oregano, salt, and pepper.
2. Rub the spice mixture evenly over both sides of the tilapia fillets.
3. Heat olive oil in a large skillet over medium-high heat.
4. Cook the tilapia for 3-4 minutes on each side, or until the fish is opaque and flakes easily with a fork.
5. Serve with lemon wedges.

(per serving):

- Calories: 180
- Protein: 23g
- Carbohydrates: 1g
- Fat: 9g
- Fiber: 0g

7. Spicy Fish Tacos

Ingredients:

- 4 white fish fillets (4 oz each, such as cod or halibut)
- 1 tbsp olive oil
- 1 tsp chili powder
- 1/2 tsp cumin
- 1/2 tsp paprika
- Salt and pepper to taste
- 8 small corn tortillas
- 1 cup shredded red cabbage
- 1/2 cup pico de gallo
- 1/4 cup low-fat sour cream
- Lime wedges for serving

Instructions:

1. Preheat the oven to 375°F (190°C).
2. In a small bowl, mix chili powder, cumin, paprika, salt, and pepper.
3. Rub the spice mixture over both sides of the fish fillets.
4. Heat olive oil in a large skillet over medium-high heat. Cook the fish for 3-4 minutes on each side, or until cooked through.
5. Warm the tortillas in the oven for 2-3 minutes.
6. Assemble the tacos by placing the fish in the tortillas and topping with shredded cabbage, pico de gallo, and a dollop of sour cream.
7. Serve with lime wedges.

(per serving):

- Calories: 250
- Protein: 21g
- Carbohydrates: 24g

- Fat: 9g
- Fiber: 3g

8. Baked Lemon Garlic Butter Shrimp

Ingredients:

- 1 lb large shrimp, peeled and deveined
- 3 tbsp unsalted butter, melted
- 3 cloves garlic, minced
- Juice of 1 lemon
- 1 tbsp chopped fresh parsley
- Salt and pepper to taste

Instructions:

1. Preheat the oven to 400°F (200°C).
2. In a baking dish, combine melted butter, garlic, lemon juice, parsley, salt, and pepper.
3. Add the shrimp and toss to coat.
4. Bake for 8-10 minutes, or until the shrimp are pink and cooked through.

5. Serve immediately.

(per serving):

- Calories: 170
- Protein: 23g
- Carbohydrates: 2g
- Fat: 8g
- Fiber: 0g

9. Cilantro Lime Grilled Mahi Mahi

Ingredients:

- 4 mahi mahi fillets (4 oz each)
- 2 tbsp olive oil
- Juice of 2 limes
- 1/4 cup chopped fresh cilantro
- 2 cloves garlic, minced
- Salt and pepper to taste

Instructions:

1. In a small bowl, mix olive oil, lime juice, cilantro, garlic, salt, and pepper.
2. Marinate the mahi mahi fillets in the mixture for 15-20 minutes.
3. Preheat the grill to medium-high heat.
4. Grill the fillets for 4-5 minutes on each side, or until the fish is opaque and flakes easily with a fork.
5. Serve immediately, garnished with additional cilantro and lime wedges.

(per serving):

- Calories: 210
- Protein: 22g
- Carbohydrates: 2g
- Fat: 13g
- Fiber: 0g

10. Scallop and Vegetable Stir-Fry

Ingredients:

- 1 lb sea scallops
- 2 tbsp olive oil, divided
- 1 red bell pepper, sliced
- 1 yellow bell pepper, sliced
- 1 zucchini, sliced
- 1 cup snap peas
- 2 cloves garlic, minced
- 2 tbsp low-sodium soy sauce
- 1 tbsp rice vinegar
- 1 tbsp honey
- 1 tsp grated fresh ginger
- Salt and pepper to taste

Instructions:

1. Heat 1 tbsp olive oil in a large skillet or wok over medium-high heat.
2. Add the scallops and cook for 2-3 minutes on each side, or until golden and cooked through. Remove from the skillet and set aside.
3. Add the remaining olive oil to the skillet. Add bell peppers, zucchini,

snap peas, and garlic. Stir-fry for 5-7 minutes, or until the vegetables are tender-crisp.

4. In a small bowl, mix soy sauce, rice vinegar, honey, ginger, salt, and pepper.
5. Return the scallops to the skillet and pour the sauce over everything. Stir to combine and cook for an additional 1-2 minutes.
6. Serve immediately.

(per serving):

- Calories: 210
- Protein: 22g
- Carbohydrates: 12g
- Fat: 8g
- Fiber: 3g

11. **Spicy Baked Catfish**

Ingredients:

- 4 catfish fillets (4 oz each)
- 2 tbsp olive oil
- 1 tsp paprika
- 1/2 tsp cayenne pepper
- 1/2 tsp garlic powder
- 1/2 tsp onion powder
- Salt and pepper to taste
- Lemon wedges for serving

Instructions:

1. Preheat oven to 375°F (190°C).
2. In a small bowl, mix paprika, cayenne pepper, garlic powder, onion powder, salt, and pepper.
3. Brush the catfish fillets with olive oil and rub with the spice mixture.
4. Place the fillets on a baking sheet lined with parchment paper.
5. Bake for 15-20 minutes, or until the fish is cooked through and flakes easily with a fork.

6. Serve with lemon wedges.

(per serving):

- Calories: 200
- Protein: 23g
- Carbohydrates: 1g
- Fat: 12g
- Fiber: 0g

12. Garlic Parmesan Crusted Halibut

Ingredients:

- 4 halibut fillets (4 oz each)
- 1/4 cup grated Parmesan cheese
- 1/4 cup breadcrumbs
- 2 cloves garlic, minced
- 2 tbsp chopped fresh parsley
- 2 tbsp olive oil
- Salt and pepper to taste

Instructions:

1. Preheat oven to 400°F (200°C).
2. In a small bowl, combine Parmesan cheese, breadcrumbs, garlic, parsley, salt, and pepper.
3. Brush the halibut fillets with olive oil and press the Parmesan mixture onto the top of each fillet.
4. Place the fillets on a baking sheet lined with parchment paper.
5. Bake for 12-15 minutes, or until the fish is cooked through and the crust is golden brown.
6. Serve immediately.

(per serving):

- Calories: 260
- Protein: 26g
- Carbohydrates: 6g
- Fat: 14g
- Fiber: 1g

13. **Citrus Grilled Swordfish**

Ingredients:

- 4 swordfish steaks (4 oz each)
- 2 tbsp olive oil
- Juice and zest of 1 orange
- Juice and zest of 1 lemon
- 2 cloves garlic, minced
- Salt and pepper to taste

Instructions:

1. In a small bowl, mix olive oil, orange juice, orange zest, lemon juice, lemon zest, garlic, salt, and pepper.
2. Marinate the swordfish steaks in the mixture for 15-20 minutes.
3. Preheat grill to medium-high heat.
4. Grill the swordfish for 4-5 minutes on each side, or until cooked through and grill marks appear.
5. Serve immediately, garnished with additional citrus zest if desired.

(per serving):

- Calories: 230
- Protein: 25g
- Carbohydrates: 2g
- Fat: 14g
- Fiber: 0g

14. Mango Avocado Shrimp Salad

Ingredients:

- 1 lb large shrimp, peeled and deveined
- 1 mango, diced
- 1 avocado, diced
- 1/4 red onion, thinly sliced
- 2 cups baby spinach
- 2 tbsp olive oil
- 1 tbsp fresh lime juice
- Salt and pepper to taste
- 1 tbsp chopped fresh cilantro

Instructions:

1. Bring a pot of water to a boil. Add shrimp and cook for 2-3 minutes until pink and opaque. Drain and cool.
2. In a large bowl, combine shrimp, mango, avocado, red onion, and baby spinach.
3. In a small bowl, whisk together olive oil, lime juice, salt, and pepper.
4. Pour the dressing over the salad and toss gently to combine.
5. Garnish with fresh cilantro before serving.

(per serving):

- Calories: 250
- Protein: 22g
- Carbohydrates: 12g
- Fat: 14g
- Fiber: 4g

15. **Asian Glazed Salmon**

Ingredients:

- 4 salmon fillets (4 oz each)
- 1/4 cup soy sauce
- 2 tbsp honey
- 1 tbsp rice vinegar
- 1 tbsp grated fresh ginger
- 2 cloves garlic, minced
- 1 tbsp sesame oil
- 1 tbsp chopped green onions
- 1 tsp sesame seeds

Instructions:

1. In a small bowl, mix soy sauce, honey, rice vinegar, ginger, garlic, and sesame oil.
2. Marinate the salmon fillets in the mixture for 15-20 minutes.
3. Preheat a grill or grill pan to medium-high heat.

4. Grill the salmon for 4-5 minutes on each side, basting with the marinade, until the fish is cooked through and glazed.
5. Garnish with green onions and sesame seeds before serving.

(per serving):

- Calories: 280
- Protein: 23g
- Carbohydrates: 10g
- Fat: 16g
- Fiber: 0g

16. Lemon Dill Baked Trout

Ingredients:

- 4 trout fillets (4 oz each)
- 2 tbsp olive oil
- Juice and zest of 1 lemon
- 2 tbsp chopped fresh dill

- 2 cloves garlic, minced
- Salt and pepper to taste

Instructions:

1. Preheat oven to 375°F (190°C).
2. In a small bowl, mix olive oil, lemon juice, lemon zest, dill, garlic, salt, and pepper.
3. Place the trout fillets on a baking sheet lined with parchment paper. Brush the fillets with the lemon dill mixture.
4. Bake for 15-20 minutes, or until the fish is cooked through and flakes easily with a fork.
5. Serve immediately, garnished with additional dill and lemon slices.

(per serving):

- Calories: 220
- Protein: 23g
- Carbohydrates: 2g

- Fat: 14g
- Fiber: 0g

17. Chili Lime Grilled Shrimp

Ingredients:

- 1 lb large shrimp, peeled and deveined
- 2 tbsp olive oil
- Juice of 2 limes
- 1 tsp chili powder
- 1/2 tsp cumin
- 2 cloves garlic, minced
- Salt and pepper to taste
- Fresh cilantro for garnish

Instructions:

1. In a small bowl, mix olive oil, lime juice, chili powder, cumin, garlic, salt, and pepper.
2. Marinate the shrimp in the mixture for 15-20 minutes.

3. Preheat grill to medium-high heat.
4. Grill the shrimp for 2-3 minutes on each side, or until pink and opaque.
5. Garnish with fresh cilantro before serving.

(per serving):

- Calories: 180
- Protein: 23g
- Carbohydrates: 2g
- Fat: 8g
- Fiber: 0g

18. Honey Mustard Baked Salmon

Ingredients:

- 4 salmon fillets (4 oz each)
- 2 tbsp Dijon mustard
- 1 tbsp honey
- 1 tbsp olive oil
- 1 tbsp chopped fresh parsley

- Salt and pepper to taste

Instructions:

1. Preheat oven to 400°F (200°C).
2. In a small bowl, mix Dijon mustard, honey, olive oil, parsley, salt, and pepper.
3. Place the salmon fillets on a baking sheet lined with parchment paper. Brush the fillets with the honey mustard mixture.
4. Bake for 12-15 minutes, or until the fish is cooked through and flakes easily with a fork.
5. Serve immediately.

(per serving):

- Calories: 260
- Protein: 23g
- Carbohydrates: 6g
- Fat: 16g

- Fiber: 0g

19. **Pesto Zucchini Shrimp**

Ingredients:

- 1 lb large shrimp, peeled and deveined
- 2 medium zucchinis, spiralized
- 2 tbsp olive oil
- 1/4 cup pesto
- 2 cloves garlic, minced
- Salt and pepper to taste
- 1/4 cup grated Parmesan cheese

Instructions:

1. Heat olive oil in a large skillet over medium-high heat.
2. Add garlic and cook for 1 minute until fragrant.
3. Add shrimp and cook for 2-3 minutes on each side until pink and opaque.

Remove shrimp from the skillet and set aside.

4. In the same skillet, add spiralized zucchini and cook for 2-3 minutes until tender.
5. Add pesto and cooked shrimp to the skillet, tossing to combine.
6. Season with salt and pepper to taste and sprinkle with Parmesan cheese before serving.

(per serving):

- Calories: 250
- Protein: 23g
- Carbohydrates: 7g
- Fat: 14g
- Fiber: 2g

20. Mediterranean Grilled Swordfish

Ingredients:

- 4 swordfish steaks (4 oz each)
- 2 tbsp olive oil
- Juice of 1 lemon
- 2 cloves garlic, minced
- 1 tsp dried oregano
- 1 tsp dried thyme
- Salt and pepper to taste
- 1/4 cup chopped fresh parsley for garnish

Instructions:

1. In a small bowl, mix olive oil, lemon juice, minced garlic, oregano, thyme, salt, and pepper to create a marinade.
2. Place the swordfish steaks in a shallow dish and pour the marinade over them. Ensure each steak is coated evenly. Let them marinate for 30 minutes in the refrigerator.
3. Preheat the grill to medium-high heat.

4. Remove the swordfish from the marinade and discard any excess marinade.
5. Grill the swordfish steaks for 4-5 minutes on each side, or until they are cooked through and have grill marks.
6. Transfer the grilled swordfish to a serving platter and garnish with chopped fresh parsley.
7. Serve hot with your favorite sides, such as grilled vegetables or a Mediterranean salad.

(per serving):

- Calories: 280
- Protein: 26g
- Carbohydrates: 2g
- Fat: 18g
- Fiber: 1g

1. **Grilled Chicken Caprese Salad**

Ingredients:

- 4 boneless, skinless chicken breasts
- 2 tablespoons olive oil
- 1 teaspoon Italian seasoning
- Salt and pepper to taste
- 4 cups mixed greens
- 1 cup cherry tomatoes, halved
- 8 ounces fresh mozzarella, sliced
- 2 tablespoons balsamic glaze

Instructions

1. Brush chicken breasts with olive oil and season with Italian seasoning, salt, and pepper.
2. Grill chicken until cooked through, about 6-8 minutes per side.
3. Arrange mixed greens on a platter and top with grilled chicken, cherry tomatoes, and mozzarella slices.
4. Drizzle with balsamic glaze and serve.

(per serving):

Calories: 290, Protein: 35g, Carbs: 8g, Fat: 13g

2. Turkey Taco Lettuce Wraps

Ingredients:

- 1 pound lean ground turkey
- 1 packet taco seasoning
- 1/2 cup water
- 8 large lettuce leaves
- 1 cup diced tomatoes
- 1/2 cup shredded low-fat cheddar cheese
- 2 tablespoons sliced black olives
- 2 tablespoons diced red onion
- 2 tablespoons chopped cilantro

Instructions

1. In a skillet, cook ground turkey over medium-high heat until browned and crumbled.
2. Add taco seasoning and water. Simmer for 5 minutes.
3. Spoon the turkey mixture into lettuce leaves.

4. Top with tomatoes, cheese, olives, onion, and cilantro.

(per serving):
Calories: 180, Protein: 20g, Carbs: 8g, Fat: 7g

3. **Lemon Garlic Roasted Chicken**

Ingredients:

- 4 boneless, skinless chicken breasts
- 2 tablespoons olive oil
- 2 cloves garlic, minced
- Zest and juice of 1 lemon
- 1 teaspoon dried thyme
- Salt and pepper to taste
- 2 cups steamed broccoli

Instructions

1. Preheat oven to 400°F (200°C).
2. In a baking dish, combine olive oil, garlic, lemon zest, lemon juice, thyme, salt, and pepper.
3. Add chicken breasts and toss to coat.
4. Bake for 25-30 minutes, or until chicken is cooked through.

5. Serve with steamed broccoli.

(per serving):
Calories: 220, Protein: 30g, Carbs: 5g, Fat:
8g

4. Turkey Meatballs with Zucchini Noodles

Ingredients:
- 1 pound lean ground turkey
- 1/2 cup breadcrumbs
- 1 egg
- 1/4 cup grated Parmesan cheese
- 2 tablespoons chopped parsley
- 1 teaspoon garlic powder
- Salt and pepper to taste
- 2 zucchinis, spiralized or julienned
- 1 cup marinara sauce

Instructions
1. Preheat oven to 375°F (190°C).
2. In a bowl, mix together ground turkey, breadcrumbs, egg, Parmesan, parsley, garlic powder, salt, and pepper.

3. Form the mixture into meatballs and place on a baking sheet.
4. Bake for 20-25 minutes, or until cooked through.
5. In a skillet, sauté zucchini noodles until tender.
6. Serve meatballs with zucchini noodles and marinara sauce.

(per serving):
Calories: 280, Protein: 25g, Carbs: 18g, Fat: 12g

5. Honey Mustard Chicken Salad

Ingredients:
- 4 boneless, skinless chicken breasts
- 2 tablespoons honey
- 2 tablespoons Dijon mustard
- 1 tablespoon olive oil
- Salt and pepper to taste
- 6 cups mixed greens
- 1 cucumber, sliced
- 1 cup cherry tomatoes, halved
- 2 tablespoons balsamic vinegar

Instructions

1. Preheat oven to 400°F (200°C).
2. In a baking dish, combine honey, mustard, olive oil, salt, and pepper.
3. Add chicken breasts and toss to coat.
4. Bake for 25-30 minutes, or until cooked through.
5. Arrange mixed greens, cucumber, and tomatoes on a platter.
6. Slice chicken and place over the salad.
7. Drizzle with balsamic vinegar and serve.

(per serving):
Calories: 280, Protein: 35g, Carbs: 12g, Fat: 9g

6. **Slow Cooker Salsa Chicken**

Ingredients:

- 4 boneless, skinless chicken breasts
- 1 cup salsa
- 1/2 cup low-sodium chicken broth
- 1 teaspoon cumin
- 1 teaspoon chili powder
- Salt and pepper to taste

- 4 cups cauliflower rice

Instructions

1. Place chicken breasts in a slow cooker.
2. Add salsa, chicken broth, cumin, chili powder, salt, and pepper.
3. Cook on low for 6-8 hours, or until chicken is cooked through.
4. Shred the chicken with two forks.
5. Serve with cauliflower rice.

(per serving):
Calories: 220, Protein: 30g, Carbs: 10g, Fat: 4g

7. **Grilled Chicken Fajita Bowls**

Ingredients:

- 4 boneless, skinless chicken breasts
- 1 tablespoon fajita seasoning
- 1 red bell pepper, sliced
- 1 yellow onion, sliced
- 2 cups cooked brown rice
- 1/2 cup salsa
- 1/4 cup low-fat sour cream
- 2 tablespoons chopped cilantro

Instructions

1. Rub chicken breasts with fajita seasoning.
2. Grill chicken, peppers, and onions until cooked through.
3. Slice the grilled chicken.
4. In a bowl, layer brown rice, grilled chicken, peppers, and onions.
5. Top with salsa, sour cream, and cilantro.

(per serving):
Calories: 330, Protein: 35g, Carbs: 35g, Fat: 6g

8. Baked Chicken Parmesan

Ingredients:
- 4 boneless, skinless chicken breasts
- 1 egg, beaten
- 1/2 cup breadcrumbs
- 1/4 cup grated Parmesan cheese
- 1 teaspoon Italian seasoning
- Salt and pepper to taste
- 1 cup marinara sauce

- 1/2 cup shredded mozzarella cheese

Instructions

1. Preheat oven to 375°F (190°C).
2. In a shallow dish, combine breadcrumbs, Parmesan, Italian seasoning, salt, and pepper.
3. Dip chicken breasts in beaten egg, then coat with breadcrumb mixture.
4. Place chicken in a baking dish and bake for 25-30 minutes.
5. Top with marinara sauce and mozzarella cheese.
6. Bake for an additional 5 minutes, or until cheese is melted.

(per serving):
Calories: 320, Protein: 35g, Carbs: 20g, Fat: 10g

9. Turkey Burger Lettuce Wraps

Ingredients:

- 1 lb lean ground turkey
- 1/4 cup finely diced onion

- 2 cloves garlic, minced
- 1 tsp dried parsley
- Salt and pepper to taste
- 8 large lettuce leaves
- Toppings: tomato, avocado, etc.

Instructions

1. In a bowl, mix together turkey, onion, garlic, parsley, salt and pepper.
2. Form into 4 patties.
3. Grill or pan fry patties until cooked through, about 5 mins per side.
4. Serve patties wrapped in lettuce leaves with desired toppings.

(Per Serving):

Calories: 220, Protein: 26g, Carbs: 4g, Fat: 11g

10. Buffalo Chicken Lettuce Wraps

Ingredients:

- 1 lb boneless skinless chicken breasts, cooked and shredded
- 1/2 cup hot sauce
- 1 tbsp butter

- 8 large lettuce leaves
- Toppings: blue cheese dressing, celery, etc.

Instructions

1. In a skillet, toss the shredded chicken with hot sauce and butter until coated.
2. Spoon buffalo chicken mixture into lettuce leaves.
3. Top with blue cheese dressing, celery, etc. if desired.

(Per Serving):
Calories: 160, Protein: 26g, Carbs: 3g, Fat: 5g

11. Chicken Sausage Skewers

Ingredients:

- 12 oz chicken sausage, sliced
- 1 red bell pepper, cut into chunks
- 1 green bell pepper, cut into chunks
- 1 red onion, cut into chunks
- Olive oil cooking spray

Instructions

1. Preheat grill or grill pan to medium-high heat.
2. Thread sausage, peppers and onions alternately onto skewers.
3. Coat skewers with cooking spray.
4. Grill for 12-15 minutes, turning occasionally, until sausage is heated through.

(Per Serving):
Calories: 200, Protein: 16g, Carbs: 8g, Fat: 10g

13. **Grilled Lemon Herb Chicken Kabobs**

Ingredients:
- 1 lb boneless skinless chicken breasts, cubed
- 1 zucchini, sliced into rounds
- 1 red onion, cut into chunks
- 2 tbsp olive oil
- 2 tbsp lemon juice
- 1 tsp dried oregano
- 1/4 tsp salt

- 1/4 tsp pepper

Instructions

1. In a bowl, toss chicken, zucchini and onion with oil, lemon juice, oregano, salt and pepper.
2. Thread onto skewers.
3. Grill for 12-15 minutes, turning occasionally, until chicken is cooked through.

(Per Serving):
Calories: 190, Protein: 25g, Carbs: 8g, Fat: 7g

14. Caprese Chicken

Ingredients:
- 4 boneless skinless chicken breasts
- 2 cups cherry tomatoes, halved
- 8 oz fresh mozzarella, sliced
- 1/4 cup fresh basil leaves
- 2 tbsp balsamic glaze
- Salt and pepper to taste

Instructions

1. Season chicken with salt and pepper
   and grill or bake until cooked through.
2. Top each chicken breast with
   tomatoes, mozzarella slices and basil
   leaves.
3. Drizzle with balsamic glaze.

(Per Serving):
Calories: 310, Protein: 41g, Carbs: 8g, Fat:
13g

15. Spinach Feta Stuffed Chicken

Ingredients:
- 4 boneless skinless chicken breasts
- 5 oz frozen chopped spinach, thawed and drained
- 1/4 cup crumbled feta
- 1 clove garlic, minced
- 1 egg, beaten
- 1/4 cup breadcrumbs
- Olive oil cooking spray

Instructions
1. Pound chicken to 1/4 inch thickness. Season with salt and pepper.

2. In a bowl, mix spinach, feta, garlic and egg.
3. Spoon spinach mixture onto chicken breasts, roll up and secure with toothpicks.
4. Coat with breadcrumbs and cooking spray.
5. Bake at 375°F for 25-30 mins until chicken is cooked through.

(Per Serving):
Calories: 250, Protein: 36g, Carbs: 10g, Fat: 7g

16. **Cajun Turkey Lettuce Wraps**

Ingredients:
- 1 lb ground turkey breast
- 1 tbsp Cajun seasoning
- 8 large lettuce leaves
- Toppings: diced tomatoes, avocado, etc.

Instructions

1. In a skillet, cook the ground turkey over medium-high heat until browned and crumbled. Drain excess fat.
2. Stir in Cajun seasoning.
3. Spoon turkey mixture into lettuce leaves and top with desired toppings.

(Per Serving):
Calories: 115, Protein: 20g, Carbs: 2g, Fat: 3g

17. Balsamic Mustard Grilled Chicken

Ingredients:
- 4 boneless, skinless chicken breasts
- 2 tbsp balsamic vinegar
- 2 tbsp Dijon mustard
- 1 tbsp olive oil
- 1 clove garlic, minced
- Salt and pepper to taste

Instructions:
1. In a bowl, whisk together the vinegar, mustard, olive oil, garlic, salt and pepper.

2. Add chicken and marinate for 30 mins to 1 hour.

3. Grill chicken until cooked through, about 6-8 mins per side, basting with marinade.

(Per Serving):
Calories: 210, Protein: 34g, Carbs: 4g, Fat: 6g

18. Thai Peanut Chicken Lettuce Cups

Ingredients:
- 1 lb ground chicken
- 2 cloves garlic, minced
- 1 tbsp grated ginger
- 3 tbsp peanut butter
- 2 tbsp soy sauce
- 1 tbsp rice vinegar
- 1 tbsp lime juice
- 8 lettuce leaves
- Toppings: shredded carrots, chopped peanuts

Instructions

1. Cook the ground chicken, garlic and ginger in a skillet until chicken is browned.
2. Stir in peanut butter, soy sauce, vinegar and lime juice.
3. Spoon chicken mixture into lettuce cups and top with carrots, peanuts, etc.

(Per Serving):
Calories: 270, Protein: 25g, Carbs: 9g, Fat: 15g

19. Spicy Chicken Meal Prep Bowls

Ingredients:
- 1 lb boneless skinless chicken breasts, diced
- 1 tbsp taco seasoning
- 2 cups cooked quinoa
- 1 cup black beans, rinsed and drained
- 1 cup corn kernels
- 1/2 cup salsa

Instructions

1. Season diced chicken with taco seasoning and cook in a skillet until browned.
2. Divide quinoa, black beans, corn and chicken between 4 meal prep containers.
3. Top each with 2 tbsp salsa.

(Per Serving):
Calories: 340, Protein: 30

20. Turkey Stuffed Peppers

Ingredients:
- 1 lb lean ground turkey
- 1/2 cup cooked brown rice
- 1 egg, beaten
- 1/4 cup finely chopped onion
- 2 cloves garlic, minced
- 1 tsp Italian seasoning
- 1/2 tsp salt
- 1/4 tsp black pepper
- 4 bell peppers, halved lengthwise and seeded
- 1 cup marinara sauce

Instructions

1. Preheat oven to 375°F.
2. In a bowl, mix together turkey, rice, egg, onion, garlic, Italian seasoning, salt and pepper until well combined.
3. Fill each pepper half with the turkey mixture.
4. Arrange peppers in a baking dish and pour marinara sauce over top.
5. Cover with foil and bake for 50-60 minutes until peppers are tender.

(Per Serving: 1 Stuffed Pepper Half):
Calories: 210, Protein: 20g, Carbs: 18g, Fat: 6g

21. Teriyaki Chicken Stir Fry

Ingredients:

- 1 lb boneless, skinless chicken breasts, cut into 1-inch pieces
- 2 tbsp low-sodium teriyaki sauce
- 2 tsp sesame oil
- 2 cups broccoli florets
- 1 red bell pepper, sliced

- 1/2 onion, sliced
- 2 cloves garlic, minced
- Salt and pepper to taste
- 2 cups cooked brown rice

Instructions

1. In a large skillet or wok, heat the sesame oil over medium-high heat.
2. Add the chicken and teriyaki sauce and stir-fry for 2-3 minutes.
3. Add the broccoli, bell pepper, onion and garlic. Season with salt and pepper.
4. Stir-fry for 5-7 minutes until chicken is cooked through and veggies are tender-crisp.
5. Serve over cooked brown rice.

(Per Serving):
Calories: 320, Protein: 30g, Carbs: 35g, Fat: 7g

1. **Caprese Skewers**

Ingredients:

1. Cherry tomatoes, fresh basil leaves, mini mozzarella balls, balsamic glaze.

Instructions:

Thread cherry tomatoes, basil leaves, and mini mozzarella balls onto skewers. Drizzle with balsamic glaze.

per skewer: Calories 50, Protein 3g, Carbs 3g, Fat 3g

Baked Zucchini Fries

Ingredients:

Zucchini, whole-wheat breadcrumbs, Parmesan cheese, egg white, salt, pepper.

Instructions:

Cut zucchini into fry shapes, dip in egg white, coat with breadcrumb-Parmesan mixture, and bake until golden brown.
 per serving (10 fries): Calories 120, Protein 6g, Carbs 16g, Fat 3g

Cucumber Bites with Tzatziki

Ingredients:

 English cucumber, Greek yogurt, lemon juice, dill, garlic, salt, pepper.

Instructions:

Slice cucumber into rounds. Mix yogurt, lemon juice, dill, garlic, salt, and pepper for tzatziki. Top cucumber rounds with tzatziki.

per serving (5 bites): Calories 60, Protein 4g, Carbs 4g, Fat 2g

Roasted Chickpeas

Ingredients:

Canned chickpeas, olive oil, smoked paprika, salt.
Instructions:

Drain and rinse chickpeas, toss with olive oil, smoked paprika, and salt. Roast in oven until crispy.

per serving (1/4 cup): Calories 120, Protein 5g, Carbs 15g, Fat 4g

Guacamole Boats

Ingredients:

Mini bell peppers, avocado, lime juice, red onion, cilantro, salt, pepper.

Instructions:

Scoop out guacamole mixture into mini bell pepper halves.

per serving (2 boats): Calories 100, Protein 2g, Carbs 8g, Fat 7g

Shrimp Cocktail

Ingredients:

Cooked shrimp, cocktail sauce, lemon wedges.

Instructions:

Serve chilled cooked shrimp with cocktail sauce and lemon wedges.

per serving (5 shrimp with sauce): Calories 80, Protein 15g, Carbs 5g, Fat 1g

Greek Salad Skewers

Ingredients:
Cherry tomatoes, cucumber, red onion, feta cheese, olives, Greek salad dressing.

Instructions:

Thread cherry tomatoes, cucumber, red onion, feta cheese, and olives onto skewers. Serve with Greek salad dressing for dipping.

per serving (2 skewers): Calories 120, Protein 5g, Carbs 6g, Fat 8g

Ingredients:

Hard-boiled eggs, Greek yogurt, Dijon mustard, dill, salt, pepper.

Instructions:

Cut hard-boiled eggs in half lengthwise, remove yolks. Mash yolks with Greek yogurt, Dijon mustard, dill, salt, and pepper. Pipe or spoon filling into egg whites.

per serving (2 deviled eggs): Calories 100, Protein 6g, Carbs 2g, Fat 7g

Hummus with Veggies

Ingredients:

Store-bought or homemade hummus, carrots, celery, bell peppers, cucumber.

Instructions:

Serve hummus with assorted fresh veggies for dipping.

per serving (1/4 cup hummus with veggies): Calories 150, Protein 5g, Carbs 17g, Fat 7g

Apple Slices with Nut Butter

Ingredients:
Apples, natural peanut or almond butter.

Instructions: Slice apples and serve with a small portion of natural nut butter for dipping.

per serving (1 apple with 2 Tbsp nut butter): Calories 200, Protein 5g, Carbs 25g, Fat 12g

Turkey Rollups

Ingredients:

Sliced deli turkey, cream cheese, spinach or sundried tomatoes.

Instructions:

Spread a thin layer of cream cheese on turkey slices, top with spinach or sundried tomatoes, and roll up.

per rollup: Calories 50, Protein 6g, Carbs 1g, Fat 3g

Tuna Stuffed Tomatoes

Ingredients:

Cherry tomatoes, canned tuna, Greek yogurt, lemon juice, dill, salt, pepper.

Instructions:

Cut tops off cherry tomatoes and scoop out insides. Mix tuna with Greek yogurt, lemon juice, dill, salt, and pepper. Stuff mixture into tomatoes.

per serving (2 stuffed tomatoes): Calories 80, Protein 10g, Carbs 4g, Fat 2g

Avocado Toast Bites

Ingredients:

Whole-wheat bread, avocado, lemon juice, salt, pepper, cherry tomatoes.

Instructions:

Mash avocado with lemon juice, salt, and pepper. Toast bread, top with avocado mixture and cherry tomato halves.

per serving (2 bites): Calories 120, Protein 4g, Carbs 15g, Fat 6g

Edamame Guacamole

Ingredients:

Edamame, avocado, lime juice, cilantro, jalapeño, salt.

Instructions:

Mash edamame and avocado with lime juice, cilantro, jalapeño, and salt. Serve with cucumber or bell pepper slices.

per serving (1/4 cup): Calories 100, Protein 5g, Carbs 6g, Fat 7g

Spicy Roasted Chickpeas

Ingredients:
Canned chickpeas, olive oil, chili powder, cumin, salt.

Instructions:
Drain and rinse chickpeas, toss with olive oil, chili powder, cumin, and salt. Roast in oven until crispy.

per serving (1/4 cup): Calories 130, Protein 5g, Carbs 15g, Fat 5g

Veggie Sushi Rolls

Ingredients:

Nori sheets, brown rice, carrots, cucumber, avocado, sesame seeds.

Instructions:

Roll up sliced veggies and brown rice in nori sheets. Sprinkle with sesame seeds.

per roll: Calories 150, Protein 3g, Carbs 28g, Fat 4g

Baked Kale Chips

Ingredients:

Kale, olive oil, salt.
Instructions:

Tear kale into bite-sized pieces, toss with olive oil and salt. Bake until crispy.

per serving (1 cup): Calories 110, Protein 4g, Carbs 9g, Fat 7g

Cottage Cheese with Fruit

Ingredients:
Low-fat cottage cheese, fresh berries or fruit.

Instructions:

Top cottage cheese with fresh berries or sliced fruit.

per serving (1/2 cup cottage cheese with 1/2 cup fruit): Calories 120, Protein 14g, Carbs 16g, Fat 1g

Cauliflower Buffalo Bites

Ingredients:

Cauliflower florets, egg, whole-wheat breadcrumbs, hot sauce.

Instructions:

Dip cauliflower in egg, coat with breadcrumbs. Bake and toss with hot sauce.

per serving (1/2 cup): Calories 100, Protein 5g, Carbs 15g, Fat 2g

Grilled Shrimp Skewers

Ingredients:

Shrimp, lime juice, garlic, cilantro, salt, pepper.

Instructions:

Marinate shrimp in lime juice, garlic, cilantro, salt, and pepper. Thread onto skewers and grill.

per skewer (5 shrimp): Calories 80, Protein 16g, Carbs 1g, Fat 1g

1. **Greek Salad**

Ingredients:
- 1 cucumber, diced
- 2 tomatoes, diced
- 1/2 red onion, thinly sliced
- 1/2 cup kalamata olives, pitted
- 4 oz feta cheese, crumbled
- 2 tbsp olive oil
- 2 tbsp red wine vinegar
- 1 tsp dried oregano
- Salt and pepper to taste

Instructions
1. In a large bowl, combine cucumber, tomatoes, onion, olives, and feta.
2. In a small bowl, whisk together olive oil, vinegar, oregano, salt, and pepper.
3. Pour the dressing over the salad and toss gently to combine.

(per serving):
Calories: 190, Fat: 14g, Carbs: 10g, Protein: 6g, Fiber: 2g

2. Spinach Strawberry Salad

Ingredients:
- 6 cups baby spinach
- 1 cup fresh strawberries, sliced
- 1/4 cup sliced almonds
- 2 oz feta cheese, crumbled
- 2 tbsp balsamic vinegar
- 1 tbsp olive oil
- 1 tsp honey
- Salt and pepper to taste

Instructions
1. In a large bowl, combine spinach, strawberries, almonds, and feta.
2. In a small bowl, whisk together balsamic vinegar, olive oil, honey, salt, and pepper.
3. Pour the dressing over the salad and toss gently to combine.

(per serving):

Calories: 150, Fat: 10g, Carbs: 10g, Protein: 5g, Fiber: 3g

3. **Chicken Caesar Salad**

Ingredients:
- 4 cups romaine lettuce, chopped
- 2 grilled chicken breasts, sliced
- 1/4 cup grated Parmesan cheese
- 1/4 cup croutons
- 2 tbsp Caesar dressing

Instructions
1. In a large bowl, combine romaine lettuce, sliced chicken, Parmesan cheese, and croutons.
2. Drizzle with Caesar dressing and toss gently to combine.

(per serving):
Calories: 250, Fat: 12g, Carbs: 10g, Protein: 26g, Fiber: 2g

4. **Taco Salad**

Ingredients:
- 4 cups romaine lettuce, chopped

- 1 cup cooked ground turkey or beef
- 1/2 cup diced tomatoes
- 1/4 cup sliced black olives
- 1/4 cup shredded cheddar cheese
- 2 tbsp salsa
- 2 tbsp low-fat sour cream

Instructions

1. In a large bowl, combine romaine lettuce, cooked meat, tomatoes, olives, and cheddar cheese.
2. Top with salsa and sour cream.

(per serving):
Calories: 250, Fat: 12g, Carbs: 10g, Protein: 20g, Fiber: 3g

5. Cobb Salad

Ingredients:

- 4 cups romaine lettuce, chopped
- 2 hard-boiled eggs, sliced
- 4 slices turkey bacon, cooked and crumbled
- 1/2 avocado, diced
- 1/4 cup diced tomatoes

- 2 tbsp blue cheese dressing

Instructions

1. In a large bowl, combine romaine lettuce, sliced eggs, crumbled bacon, avocado, and tomatoes.
2. Drizzle with blue cheese dressing and toss gently to combine.

(per serving):
Calories: 300, Fat: 20g, Carbs: 10g, Protein: 18g, Fiber: 5g

6. **Quinoa Salad with Roasted Veggies**

Ingredients:

- 1 cup cooked quinoa
- 1 cup roasted vegetables (e.g., bell peppers, zucchini, onion)
- 1/4 cup feta cheese
- 2 tbsp olive oil
- 2 tbsp lemon juice
- Salt and pepper to taste

Instructions

1. In a large bowl, combine cooked quinoa, roasted vegetables, and feta cheese.
2. In a small bowl, whisk together olive oil, lemon juice, salt, and pepper.
3. Pour the dressing over the salad and toss gently to combine.

(per serving):
Calories: 250, Fat: 14g, Carbs: 22g, Protein: 8g, Fiber: 4g

7. Caprese Salad

Ingredients:
- 2 cups cherry tomatoes, halved
- 8 oz fresh mozzarella cheese, sliced
- 1/4 cup fresh basil leaves
- 2 tbsp balsamic vinegar
- 1 tbsp olive oil
- Salt and pepper to taste

Instructions
1. In a large bowl, combine cherry tomatoes, mozzarella cheese, and basil leaves.

2. In a small bowl, whisk together balsamic vinegar, olive oil, salt, and pepper.
3. Pour the dressing over the salad and toss gently to combine.

(per serving):
Calories: 200, Fat: 14g, Carbs: 6g, Protein: 12g, Fiber: 1g

8. Waldorf Salad

Ingredients:
- 2 cups diced apples
- 1/2 cup diced celery
- 1/4 cup walnuts
- 1/4 cup non-fat Greek yogurt
- 1 tbsp lemon juice
- 1 tsp honey
- Salt and pepper to taste

Instructions
1. In a large bowl, combine diced apples, celery, and walnuts.

2. In a small bowl, whisk together Greek yogurt, lemon juice, honey, salt, and pepper.
3. Pour the dressing over the salad and toss gently to combine.

(per serving):
Calories: 150, Fat: 8g, Carbs: 18g, Protein: 3g, Fiber: 3g

9. Lentil Salad

Ingredients:
- 1 cup cooked lentils
- 1 cup diced cucumber
- 1/2 cup diced tomatoes
- 1/4 cup diced red onion
- 2 tbsp lemon juice
- 1 tbsp olive oil
- Salt and pepper to taste

Instructions
1. In a large bowl, combine cooked lentils, cucumber, tomatoes, and red onion.

2. In a small bowl, whisk together lemon juice, olive oil, salt, and pepper.

3. Pour the dressing over the salad and toss gently to combine.

(per serving):

Calories: 200, Fat: 6g, Carbs: 28g, Protein: 10g, Fiber: 10g

10. **Asian Slaw**

Ingredients:

- 3 cups shredded cabbage
- 1 cup shredded carrots
- 1/4 cup sliced green onions
- 2 tbsp rice vinegar
- 1 tbsp sesame oil
- 1 tsp honey
- Salt and pepper to taste

Instructions

1. In a large bowl, combine shredded cabbage, carrots, and green onions.

2. In a small bowl, whisk together rice vinegar, sesame oil, honey, salt, and pepper.

3. Pour the dressing over the slaw and toss gently to combine.

(per serving):
Calories: 100, Fat: 4g, Carbs: 14g, Protein: 2g, Fiber: 3g

11. Kale and Quinoa Salad

Ingredients:
- 4 cups kale, stems removed and chopped
- 1 cup cooked quinoa
- 1/2 cup diced cucumber
- 1/4 cup crumbled feta cheese
- 2 tbsp lemon juice
- 1 tbsp olive oil
- Salt and pepper to taste

Instructions
1. In a large bowl, combine kale, quinoa, cucumber, and feta cheese.
2. In a small bowl, whisk together lemon juice, olive oil, salt, and pepper.

3. Pour the dressing over the salad and massage into the kale to soften it. Toss to combine.

per serving: Calories 180, Fat 8g, Carbs 20g, Protein 8g, Fiber 4g

12. Southwestern Salad

Ingredients:
- 4 cups romaine lettuce, chopped
- 1 cup cooked black beans
- 1/2 cup corn kernels
- 1/4 cup diced tomatoes
- 2 tbsp diced red onion
- 2 tbsp ranch dressing
- 1 tbsp salsa

Instructions
1. In a large bowl, combine romaine lettuce, black beans, corn, tomatoes, and red onion.
2. Drizzle with ranch dressing and top with salsa.

per serving: Calories 200, Fat 7g, Carbs 28g, Protein 8g, Fiber 8g

13. **Avocado and Grapefruit Salad**

Ingredients:
- 2 cups mixed greens
- 1 grapefruit, peeled and sectioned
- 1 avocado, diced
- 2 tbsp sliced almonds
- 2 tbsp lemon juice
- 1 tbsp olive oil
- Salt and pepper to taste

Instructions
1. In a large bowl, combine mixed greens, grapefruit sections, avocado, and sliced almonds.
2. In a small bowl, whisk together lemon juice, olive oil, salt, and pepper.
3. Pour the dressing over the salad and toss gently to combine.

per serving: Calories 250, Fat 18g, Carbs 20g, Protein 4g, Fiber 8g

14. **Thai Crunch Salad**

Ingredients:
- 4 cups shredded cabbage
- 1 cup shredded carrots
- 1/2 cup sliced red bell pepper
- 1/4 cup chopped cilantro
- 2 tbsp rice vinegar
- 1 tbsp peanut butter
- 1 tsp honey
- Salt and pepper to taste

Instructions
1. In a large bowl, combine shredded cabbage, carrots, red bell pepper, and cilantro.
2. In a small bowl, whisk together rice vinegar, peanut butter, honey, salt, and pepper.
3. Pour the dressing over the salad and toss gently to combine.

per serving: Calories 120, Fat 5g, Carbs 16g, Protein 3g, Fiber 4g

15. Nicoise Salad

Ingredients:

- 4 cups mixed greens
- 1 can (5 oz) tuna, drained
- 1/2 cup steamed green beans
- 1/4 cup sliced cherry tomatoes
- 2 hard-boiled eggs, sliced
- 2 tbsp olive oil
- 1 tbsp red wine vinegar
- Salt and pepper to taste

Instructions

1. In a large bowl, combine mixed greens, tuna, green beans, cherry tomatoes, and sliced eggs.
2. In a small bowl, whisk together olive oil, red wine vinegar, salt, and pepper.
3. Pour the dressing over the salad and toss gently to combine.

per serving: Calories 250, Fat 14g, Carbs 8g, Protein 22g, Fiber 3g

16. Broccoli Salad

Ingredients:

- 4 cups broccoli florets
- 1/2 cup diced red onion
- 1/4 cup raisins
- 1/4 cup sliced almonds
- 2 tbsp non-fat Greek yogurt
- 1 tbsp apple cider vinegar
- 1 tsp Dijon mustard
- Salt and pepper to taste

Instructions

1. In a large bowl, combine broccoli florets, red onion, raisins, and sliced almonds.
2. In a small bowl, whisk together Greek yogurt, apple cider vinegar, Dijon mustard, salt, and pepper.
3. Pour the dressing over the salad and toss gently to combine.

per serving: Calories 150, Fat 6g, Carbs 20g, Protein 6g, Fiber 5g

17. Salmon Avocado Salad

Ingredients:

- 4 cups mixed greens

- 4 oz grilled salmon
- 1/2 avocado, diced
- 1/4 cup sliced cucumber
- 2 tbsp lemon juice
- 1 tbsp olive oil
- Salt and pepper to taste

Instructions

1. In a large bowl, combine mixed greens, grilled salmon, avocado, and sliced cucumber.
2. In a small bowl, whisk together lemon juice, olive oil, salt, and pepper.
3. Pour the dressing over the salad and toss gently to combine.

per serving: Calories 300, Fat 20g, Carbs 8g, Protein 24g, Fiber 5g

18. Chickpea and Feta Salad

Ingredients:

- 1 can (15 oz) chickpeas, drained and rinsed
- 1 cup diced cucumber
- 1/2 cup crumbled feta cheese

- 1/4 cup diced red onion
- 2 tbsp lemon juice
- 1 tbsp olive oil
- Salt and pepper to taste

Instructions

1. In a large bowl, combine chickpeas, cucumber, feta cheese, and red onion.
2. In a small bowl, whisk together lemon juice, olive oil, salt, and pepper.
3. Pour the dressing over the salad and toss gently to combine.

per serving: Calories 200, Fat 9g, Carbs 21g, Protein 9g, Fiber 6g

19. Shrimp and Mango Salad

Ingredients:

- 4 cups mixed greens
- 8 oz cooked shrimp, peeled and deveined
- 1 mango, diced
- 1/4 cup sliced red onion
- 2 tbsp lime juice
- 1 tbsp olive oil

- Salt and pepper to taste

Instructions

1. In a large bowl, combine mixed greens, shrimp, mango, and red onion.
2. In a small bowl, whisk together lime juice, olive oil, salt, and pepper.
3. Pour the dressing over the salad and toss gently to combine.

per serving: Calories 250, Fat 8g, Carbs 20g, Protein 24g, Fiber 4g

20. Beet and Goat Cheese Salad

Ingredients:

- 4 cups mixed greens
- 1 cup roasted beets, diced
- 2 oz goat cheese, crumbled
- 1/4 cup walnuts
- 2 tbsp balsamic vinegar
- 1 tbsp olive oil
- Salt and pepper to taste

Instructions

1. In a large bowl, combine mixed greens, roasted beets, goat cheese, and walnuts.
2. In a small bowl, whisk together balsamic vinegar, olive oil, salt, and pepper.
3. Pour the dressing over the salad and toss gently to combine.

per serving: Calories 250, Fat 18g, Carbs 16g, Protein 8g, Fiber 4g

HEALTHY RECIPES

1. Grilled Chicken Veggie Bowls

Ingredients:
- 4 grilled chicken breasts, sliced
- 2 cups cooked quinoa
- 2 cups roasted broccoli florets
- 1 cup cherry tomatoes, halved
- 1/4 cup feta cheese
- 2 tbsp lemon juice
- 1 tbsp olive oil
- Salt and pepper to taste

Instructions

1. In a large bowl, combine sliced chicken, cooked quinoa, roasted broccoli, cherry tomatoes, and feta cheese.
2. In a small bowl, whisk together lemon juice, olive oil, salt, and pepper.
3. Pour the dressing over the bowl and toss gently to combine.

(per serving):
Calories: 350, Fat: 12g, Carbs: 30g, Protein: 35g, Fiber: 6g

2. Vegetarian Chili

Ingredients:

- 1 tbsp olive oil
- 1 onion, diced
- 3 cloves garlic, minced
- 1 bell pepper, diced
- 2 cans (15 oz each) diced tomatoes
- 1 can (15 oz) black beans, drained and rinsed

- 1 can (15 oz) kidney beans, drained and rinsed
- 1 tbsp chili powder
- 1 tsp cumin
- Salt and pepper to taste

Instructions

1. In a large pot, heat olive oil over medium heat. Add onion and garlic, and cook for 2-3 minutes until fragrant.
2. Add bell pepper, diced tomatoes, black beans, kidney beans, chili powder, cumin, salt, and pepper. Stir to combine.
3. Bring to a simmer and let cook for 15-20 minutes, stirring occasionally.

(per serving):
Calories: 220, Fat: 4g, Carbs: 38g, Protein: 12g, Fiber: 12g

3. **Zucchini Noodles with Shrimp**

Ingredients:

- 4 zucchini, spiralized into noodles

- 1 lb shrimp, peeled and deveined
- 2 cloves garlic, minced
- 2 tbsp lemon juice
- 2 tbsp olive oil
- Salt and pepper to taste
- 1/4 cup grated Parmesan cheese

Instructions

1. In a large skillet, heat 1 tbsp olive oil over medium-high heat. Add shrimp and garlic, and cook until shrimp is opaque, about 3-4 minutes. Remove shrimp from skillet and set aside.
2. In the same skillet, heat remaining 1 tbsp olive oil. Add zucchini noodles and lemon juice, and cook for 2-3 minutes until slightly softened.
3. Return shrimp to the skillet, and toss everything together. Season with salt and pepper, and sprinkle with Parmesan cheese.

(per serving):
Calories: 260, Fat: 12g, Carbs: 12g, Protein: 27g, Fiber: 2g

4. Cauliflower Fried Rice

Ingredients:

- 4 cups cauliflower rice
- 1 tbsp sesame oil
- 2 eggs, beaten
- 1/2 cup frozen peas and carrots
- 2 green onions, sliced
- 2 cloves garlic, minced
- 2 tbsp low-sodium soy sauce
- Salt and pepper to taste

Instructions

1. In a large skillet, heat sesame oil over medium heat. Add beaten eggs and swirl to create a thin omelet. Once cooked, remove from skillet and slice into strips.
2. In the same skillet, add cauliflower rice, peas, carrots, green onions, and garlic. Cook for 5-7 minutes, stirring frequently, until vegetables are tender.
3. Add egg strips and soy sauce, and toss everything together. Season with salt and pepper to taste.

(per serving):
Calories: 180, Fat: 7g, Carbs: 15g, Protein: 10g, Fiber: 5g

5. Quinoa Stuffed Peppers

Ingredients:

- 4 bell peppers, halved and seeded
- 1 cup cooked quinoa
- 1 can (15 oz) black beans, drained and rinsed
- 1 cup corn kernels
- 1/2 cup salsa
- 1/4 cup grated cheddar cheese
- Salt and pepper to taste

Instructions

1. Preheat oven to 375°F (190°C).
2. In a large bowl, combine cooked quinoa, black beans, corn, salsa, and salt and pepper to taste.
3. Stuff the bell pepper halves with the quinoa mixture, and place in a baking dish.
4. Bake for 30 minutes, then top with grated cheddar cheese and bake for an

additional 5 minutes, or until the cheese is melted.

(per serving):
Calories: 280, Fat: 6g, Carbs: 46g, Protein: 13g, Fiber: 11g

6. Turkey Lettuce Wraps

Ingredients:
- 1 lb ground turkey
- 1 tbsp sesame oil
- 1 red bell pepper, diced
- 2 cloves garlic, minced
- 1 tbsp grated ginger
- 3 tbsp low-sodium soy sauce
- 1 tbsp rice vinegar
- Butter lettuce leaves
- Sliced green onions and sesame seeds (for garnish)

Instructions
1. In a large skillet, cook ground turkey over medium-high heat until browned and crumbled. Drain excess fat.

2. Add sesame oil, bell pepper, garlic, and ginger to the skillet. Cook for 2-3 minutes until fragrant.
3. Add soy sauce and rice vinegar, and stir to combine.
4. Serve the turkey mixture in lettuce leaves, and garnish with green onions and sesame seeds.

(per serving):
Calories: 250, Fat: 12g, Carbs: 8g, Protein: 27g, Fiber: 2g

7. Mediterranean Chickpea Salad

Ingredients:
- 1 can (15 oz) chickpeas, drained and rinsed
- 1 cup cherry tomatoes, halved
- 1 cucumber, diced
- 1/2 red onion, thinly sliced
- 1/4 cup crumbled feta cheese
- 2 tbsp olive oil
- 2 tbsp lemon juice
- 1 tbsp red wine vinegar

- Salt and pepper to taste

Instructions

1. In a large bowl, combine chickpeas, cherry tomatoes, cucumber, red onion, and feta cheese.
2. In a small bowl, whisk together olive oil, lemon juice, red wine vinegar, salt, and pepper.
3. Pour the dressing over the salad and toss gently to combine.

(per serving):
Calories: 220, Fat: 10g, Carbs: 24g, Protein: 8g, Fiber: 6g

8. Lentil Vegetable Soup

Ingredients:
- 1 tbsp olive oil
- 1 onion, diced
- 3 carrots, sliced
- 3 celery stalks, sliced
- 4 cloves garlic, minced
- 1 cup dried lentils
- 4 cups vegetable or chicken broth

- 2 cups baby spinach
- Salt and pepper to taste

Instructions

1. In a large pot, heat olive oil over medium heat. Add onion, carrots, celery, and garlic. Cook for 5 minutes until fragrant.
2. Add dried lentils and broth. Bring to a boil, then reduce heat and simmer for 20-25 minutes, until lentils are tender.
3. Stir in baby spinach and cook for 2 more minutes until wilted.
4. Season with salt and pepper to taste.

(per serving):
Calories: 220, Fat: 4g, Carbs: 34g, Protein: 12g, Fiber: 13g

9. Egg Roll in a Bowl

Ingredients:
- 1 lb ground turkey or chicken
- 2 tbsp sesame oil
- 1 bag (14 oz) coleslaw mix
- 2 cloves garlic, minced

- 1 tsp grated ginger
- 3 tbsp low-sodium soy sauce
- 1 tsp rice vinegar
- Salt and pepper to taste
- Sliced green onions and sesame seeds (for garnish)

Instructions

1. In a large skillet, cook ground turkey or chicken over medium-high heat until browned and crumbled. Drain excess fat.
2. Add sesame oil, coleslaw mix, garlic, and ginger to the skillet. Cook for 2-3 minutes until fragrant.
3. Add soy sauce, rice vinegar, salt, and pepper. Stir to combine.
4. Serve in bowls and garnish with green onions and sesame seeds.

(per serving):
Calories: 280, Fat: 15g, Carbs: 12g, Protein: 25g, Fiber: 3g

11. Tuna Stuffed Avocado

Ingredients:

- 2 large avocados, halved and pitted
- 1 can (5 oz) tuna, drained
- 1/4 cup diced red onion
- 1/4 cup diced tomatoes
- 2 tbsp chopped fresh cilantro
- 2 tbsp lime juice
- Salt and pepper to taste

Instructions

1. Scoop out a small amount of avocado flesh from each half, leaving a hole for the filling.
2. In a medium bowl, combine the tuna, red onion, tomatoes, cilantro, and lime juice. Season with salt and pepper to taste.
3. Stuff the tuna mixture into the avocado halves, dividing evenly.
4. Serve immediately or refrigerate until ready to eat.

(per serving):
Calories: 280

Total Fat: 19g

Carbohydrates: 13g

Fiber: 8g

Protein:18g

Day 1:

Breakfast - Avocado Toast:

2 slices whole grain bread (4 SmartPoints)

1/2 avocado, mashed (4 SmartPoints)

Sliced tomatoes and a sprinkle of black pepper

Lunch - Grilled Chicken Salad:

Grilled chicken breast (0 SmartPoints)

Mixed greens, cucumber, cherry tomatoes, and bell peppers (0 SmartPoints)

Balsamic vinaigrette dressing (2 SmartPoints)

Dinner - Baked Salmon with Roasted Vegetables:

Baked salmon fillet (0 SmartPoints)

Roasted broccoli, carrots, and cauliflower (0 SmartPoints)

Quinoa or brown rice (4 SmartPoints)

Snack - Greek Yogurt with Berries:

Non-fat Greek yogurt (2 SmartPoints)

Fresh berries (0 SmartPoints)

Day 2:

Breakfast - Veggie Omelette:

2 eggs, beaten (0 SmartPoints)

Diced bell peppers, onions, spinach, and mushrooms (0 SmartPoints)

1/4 cup reduced-fat shredded cheese (3 SmartPoints)

Lunch - Turkey and Veggie Wrap:

Whole wheat wrap (3 SmartPoints)

Sliced turkey breast (0 SmartPoints)

Lettuce, tomato, cucumber, and bell peppers (0 SmartPoints)

Mustard or hummus (1 SmartPoint)

Dinner - Turkey Chili:

Ground turkey chili with beans and vegetables (3 SmartPoints)

Side salad with mixed greens and vinaigrette dressing (2 SmartPoints)

Snack - Apple Slices with Peanut Butter:

Sliced apple (0 SmartPoints)

1 tablespoon peanut butter (3 SmartPoints)

Day 3:

Breakfast - Overnight Oats:

1/2 cup rolled oats (4 SmartPoints)

Unsweetened almond milk (1 SmartPoint)

Sliced banana and a sprinkle of cinnamon (0 SmartPoints)

Lunch - Quinoa Salad:

Quinoa (4 SmartPoints)

Cherry tomatoes, cucumber, red onion, and parsley (0 SmartPoints)

Lemon vinaigrette dressing (2 SmartPoints)

Grilled chicken breast (0 SmartPoints)

Dinner - Stir-Fried Tofu with Vegetables:

Stir-fried tofu with broccoli, bell peppers, snap peas, and carrots (3 SmartPoints)

Brown rice (4 SmartPoints)

Snack - Baby Carrots with Hummus:

Baby carrots (0 SmartPoints)

Hummus (2 SmartPoints)

Day 4:

Breakfast - Whole Grain Pancakes:

2 whole grain pancakes (4 SmartPoints)

Fresh berries and a drizzle of honey (0 SmartPoints)

Lunch - Tuna Salad Lettuce Wraps:

Tuna salad (0 SmartPoints)

Lettuce leaves for wrapping (0 SmartPoints)

Sliced cucumber and cherry tomatoes (0 SmartPoints)

Dinner - Grilled Shrimp Skewers with Quinoa Salad:

Grilled shrimp skewers (0 SmartPoints)

Quinoa salad with cherry tomatoes, cucumber, red onion, and feta cheese (6 SmartPoints)

Snack - Non-fat Greek Yogurt with Granola:

Non-fat Greek yogurt (2 SmartPoints)

1/4 cup granola (4 SmartPoints)

Day 5:

Breakfast - Scrambled Eggs with Spinach and Feta:

Scrambled eggs with spinach and feta cheese (4 SmartPoints)

Lunch - Chicken Caesar Salad:

Grilled chicken breast (0 SmartPoints)

Romaine lettuce, cherry tomatoes, and Parmesan cheese (0 SmartPoints)

Light Caesar dressing (3 SmartPoints)

Dinner - Baked Cod with Roasted Asparagus:

Baked cod fillet (0 SmartPoints)

Roasted asparagus (0 SmartPoints)

Quinoa or brown rice (4 SmartPoints)

Snack - Mixed Nuts:

1/4 cup mixed nuts (6 SmartPoints)

Day 6:

Breakfast - Berry Smoothie:

1 cup mixed berries (0 SmartPoints)

1/2 banana (0 SmartPoints)

1/2 cup non-fat Greek yogurt (2 SmartPoints)

Unsweetened almond milk (1 SmartPoint)

1 tablespoon chia seeds (3 SmartPoints)

Lunch - Turkey and Veggie Wrap:

Whole wheat wrap (3 SmartPoints)

Sliced turkey breast (0 SmartPoints)

Lettuce, tomato, cucumber, and bell peppers (0 SmartPoints)

Mustard or hummus (1 SmartPoint)

Dinner - Vegetarian Chili:

Vegetarian chili with beans, tomatoes, corn, and bell peppers (5 SmartPoints)

Side salad with mixed greens and vinaigrette dressing (2 SmartPoints)

Snack - Celery Sticks with Almond Butter:

Celery sticks (0 SmartPoints)

Almond butter (3 SmartPoints)

Day 7:

Breakfast - Greek Yogurt Parfait:

Non-fat Greek yogurt (2 SmartPoints)

Mixed berries (0 SmartPoints)

1/4 cup granola (4 SmartPoints)

Lunch - Caprese Salad:

Sliced tomatoes, fresh mozzarella, and basil (2 SmartPoints)

Drizzle with balsamic glaze (2 SmartPoints)

Grilled chicken breast (0 SmartPoints)

Dinner - Lemon Garlic Shrimp Pasta:

Whole wheat pasta (5 SmartPoints)

Lemon garlic shrimp (3 SmartPoints)

Steamed broccoli on the side (0 SmartPoints)

Snack - Air-Popped Popcorn:

2 cups air-popped popcorn (3 SmartPoints)

Day 8:

Breakfast - Spinach and Feta Egg Muffins:

- 2 spinach and feta egg muffins (4 SmartPoints)
- Sliced strawberries (0 SmartPoints)

Lunch - Turkey and Veggie Wrap:

- Whole wheat wrap (3 SmartPoints)
- Sliced turkey breast (0 SmartPoints)
- Lettuce, tomato, cucumber, and bell peppers (0 SmartPoints)
- Mustard or hummus (1 SmartPoint)

Dinner - Baked Chicken with Sweet Potato and Green Beans:

- Baked chicken breast (0 SmartPoints)
- Roasted sweet potato wedges (4 SmartPoints)
- Steamed green beans (0 SmartPoints)

Snack - Non-fat Greek Yogurt with Honey:

- Non-fat Greek yogurt (2 SmartPoints)
- Drizzle of honey (1 SmartPoint)

Day 9:

Breakfast - Whole Grain Toast with Almond Butter and Banana:

- 2 slices whole grain toast (4 SmartPoints)
- 2 tablespoons almond butter (6 SmartPoints)
- Sliced banana (0 SmartPoints)

Lunch - Mediterranean Chickpea Salad:

- Chickpeas, cucumber, cherry tomatoes, red onion, olives, and feta cheese (6 SmartPoints)
- Lemon vinaigrette dressing (2 SmartPoints)

Dinner - Grilled Salmon with Asparagus and Quinoa:

- Grilled salmon fillet (0 SmartPoints)
- Roasted asparagus (0 SmartPoints)
- Quinoa (4 SmartPoints)

Snack - Baby Carrots with Hummus:

- Baby carrots (0 SmartPoints)
- Hummus (2 SmartPoints)

Day 10:

Breakfast - Berry Protein Smoothie:

- 1 cup mixed berries (0 SmartPoints)
- 1 scoop protein powder (2 SmartPoints)
- Unsweetened almond milk (1 SmartPoint)
- Handful of spinach (0 SmartPoints)

Lunch - Turkey and Avocado Wrap:

- Whole wheat wrap (3 SmartPoints)
- Sliced turkey breast (0 SmartPoints)
- Sliced avocado (3 SmartPoints)
- Lettuce, tomato, and cucumber (0 SmartPoints)

Dinner - Veggie Stir-Fry with Tofu:

- Stir-fried tofu with mixed vegetables (4 SmartPoints)
- Brown rice (4 SmartPoints)

Snack - Apple Slices with Peanut Butter:

- Sliced apple (0 SmartPoints)
- 1 tablespoon peanut butter (3 SmartPoints)

Day 11:

Breakfast - Greek Yogurt Parfait:

- Non-fat Greek yogurt (2 SmartPoints)
- Mixed berries (0 SmartPoints)
- 1/4 cup granola (4 SmartPoints)

Lunch - Caprese Salad:

- Sliced tomatoes, fresh mozzarella, and basil (2 SmartPoints)
- Drizzle with balsamic glaze (2 SmartPoints)
- Grilled chicken breast (0 SmartPoints)

Dinner - Turkey Meatballs with Marinara Sauce and Zucchini Noodles:

- Turkey meatballs (5 SmartPoints)
- Marinara sauce (2 SmartPoints)
- Zucchini noodles (0 SmartPoints)

Snack - Air-Popped Popcorn:

- 2 cups air-popped popcorn (3 SmartPoints)

Day 12:

Breakfast - Veggie Scramble:

- Scrambled eggs with diced bell peppers, onions, spinach, and mushrooms (4 SmartPoints)

Lunch - Tuna Salad Lettuce Wraps:

- Tuna salad (0 SmartPoints)
- Lettuce leaves for wrapping (0 SmartPoints)
- Sliced cucumber and cherry tomatoes (0 SmartPoints)

Dinner - Lemon Garlic Shrimp Pasta:

- Whole wheat pasta (5 SmartPoints)
- Lemon garlic shrimp (3 SmartPoints)
- Steamed broccoli on the side (0 SmartPoints)

Snack - Mixed Nuts:

- 1/4 cup mixed nuts (6 SmartPoints)

Day 13:

Breakfast - Peanut Butter Banana Overnight Oats:

- 1/2 cup rolled oats (4 SmartPoints)
- Unsweetened almond milk (1 SmartPoint)
- 1 tablespoon peanut butter (3 SmartPoints)

- Sliced banana (0 SmartPoints)

Lunch - Chicken Caesar Salad:

- Grilled chicken breast (0 SmartPoints)
- Romaine lettuce, cherry tomatoes, and Parmesan cheese (0 SmartPoints)
- Light Caesar dressing (3 SmartPoints)

Dinner - Grilled Swordfish with Roasted Vegetables:

- Grilled swordfish steak (0 SmartPoints)
- Roasted vegetables (0 SmartPoints)
- Quinoa or brown rice (4 SmartPoints)

Snack - Celery Sticks with Almond Butter:

- Celery sticks (0 SmartPoints)
- Almond butter (3 SmartPoints)

Day 14:

Breakfast - Avocado Toast with Poached Egg:

- 2 slices whole grain bread (4 SmartPoints)
- 1/2 avocado, mashed (4 SmartPoints)
- Poached egg (0 SmartPoints)

Lunch - Turkey and Veggie Wrap:

- Whole wheat wrap (3 SmartPoints)
- Sliced turkey breast (0 SmartPoints)
- Lettuce, tomato, cucumber, and bell peppers (0 SmartPoints)

- Mustard or hummus (1 SmartPoint)

Dinner - Baked Cod with Lemon Herb Butter and Steamed Broccoli:

- Baked cod fillet (0 SmartPoints)
- Lemon herb butter sauce (3 SmartPoints)
- Steamed broccoli (0 SmartPoints)

Snack - Non-fat Greek Yogurt with Berries:

- Non-fat Greek yogurt (2 SmartPoints)
- Fresh berries (0 SmartPoints)

CONCLUSION

Embrace the vibrant flavors, treat your tastebuds, and nourish your body and soul with this transformative cookbook. Within these pages, you'll discover a world of culinary possibilities that celebrate nature's bounty, ignite your passion for cooking, and inspire you to embark on a journey of flavor exploration. Let this be the catalyst for a lifetime of delicious, wholesome, and soul-satisfying meals that will elevate your dining experiences to new heights of bliss. Unlock the secrets, awaken your senses, and embark on a flavorful adventure that will forever change the way you perceive and enjoy food.

THE END

www.ingramcontent.com/pod-product-compliance
Lightning Source LLC
Chambersburg PA
CBHW061632250726
48659CB00004B/1185